Supercharge
YOUR LIFE

eat · love · connect

How to put real food
at the heart of everything

LEE HOLMES

MURDOCH BOOKS
SYDNEY · LONDON

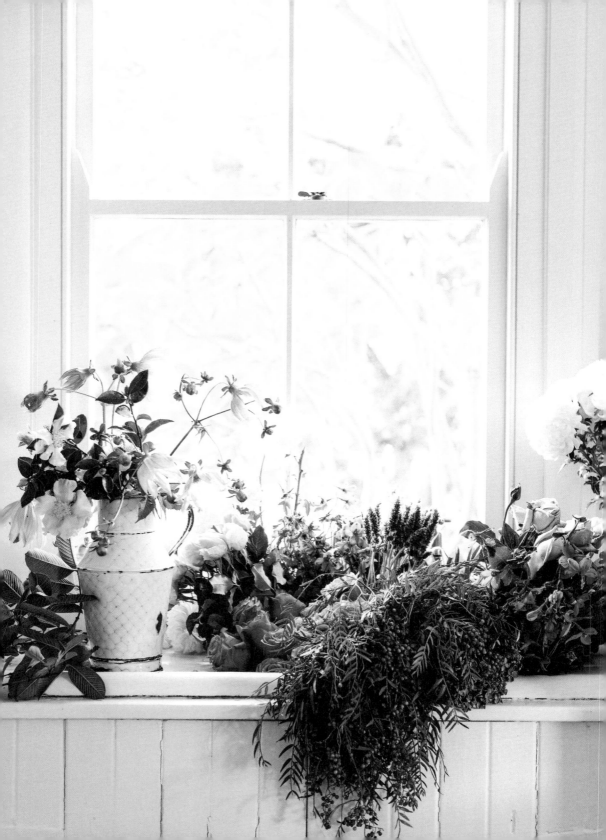

Contents

PART ONE
eat

Set up your supercharged kitchen, learn how to cook wholesome
ingredients well and enjoy nourishing, tasty recipes.

PART TWO
love

Create a warm and welcoming home, with feel-good food and great
produce — then radiate that joy out into your community.

PART THREE
connect

Make food a cause for celebration by bringing
everyone together.

eat

love

connect

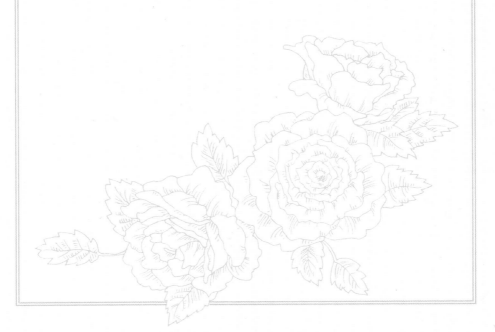

Why I wrote this book

Have you spent years on restrictive and fad diets? If so, it's time to turn the tables on forbidden fruits and sweet potato prohibitions, and allow yourself to fall in love with food all over again. I'm encouraging you to step away from the fear and move towards embracing the goodness of Mother Nature's most beautiful gifts.

The essence of life is constant growth; we're continually moving, evolving and changing. In this book, I hope to help you corral your thoughts so you can stay open to new experiences and relish change. I'm going to empower you with recipes and new ingredients that are bursting with feel-good wholesomeness and love.

True flavour doesn't come in a shiny packet or a cube.

All the recipes in *Supercharge Your Life* are hearty, wholesome and energising. It's a culmination of the knowledge I've acquired through my journey of writing books, and it ends as it begins: in the heart of my home – my supercharged kitchen, beside a purring stove.

You'll discover mouth-watering old-school recipes for pleasure and fulfilment that will steer you towards living a supercharged life. Whether you're a novice in the kitchen or cooking is second nature to you, you'll find my suggestions for flavour pairings and food partnerships invaluable when creating the delicious recipes in this book, and they'll arouse your interest in new flavours for your own creations. You'll also learn how to simplify meal preparation, and stock your pantry, fridge and freezer well.

You'll find out how to set up your enduring kitchen, outfitting it with the tools you need, from spice rack to high-speed blender. You'll discover how to simplify meal preparation. You'll master the lost art of cooking vegetables – and wave goodbye to soggy overcooked veg. You'll redefine your relationship with food and embrace commonsense eating. You may even be inspired to grow your own vegetables and herbs.

Throughout this book you'll be guided by real food and purposeful eating principles, and be enthused to recreate the lost art of mealtimes. You'll discover the beauty in simple things, and be inspired to create tablescapes that turn your house into a home and kindle sweet moments of joy, gathered around a table filled with love and sharing. You'll find food's true purpose, and discover the value of feeling at home in the kitchen – and of living a supercharged life.

The book's philosophy is based on a balanced approach, the thoughtful eating practices of Ayurveda, the anti-inflammatory and nutritional principles I follow, and the ease and simplicity of creating home-made supercharged meals with accessible and healthy ingredients.

Learn how to give up punishing yourself and fall in love with food again – and on the way rediscover the art of freedom and pleasure through beautiful and nourishing food.

Lee xo

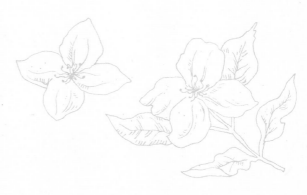

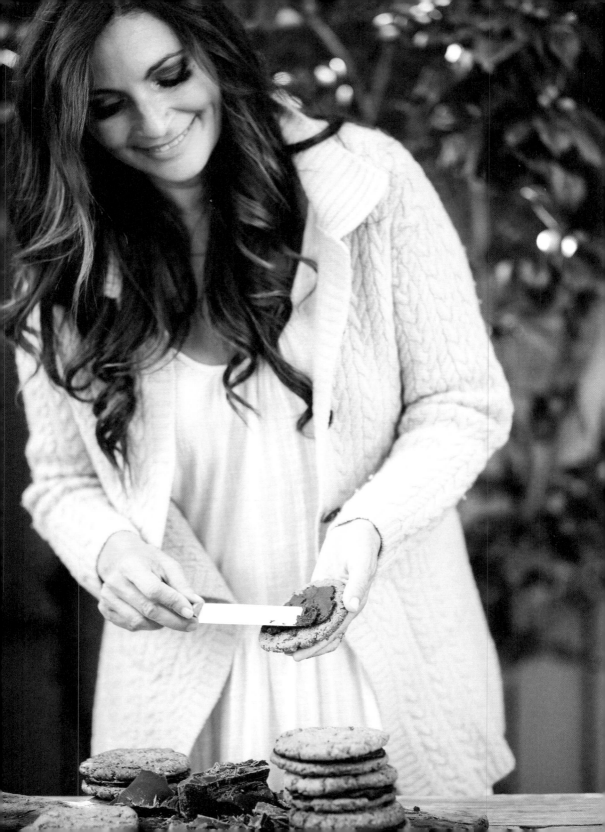

Eating from a place of freedom and pleasure

At the heart of our deep desire for pleasure and fulfilment can lie a need that's inherently driven by fear. Fear of death, fear of loss, fear of loneliness or fear of abandonment – fear has many motives and guises.

Have you ever noticed how particular industries perpetuate our fears for their own gain or satisfaction? When it comes to health and wellness, some of our current health trends can reflect this fear rather than our freedom.

FREEDOM

{ FREEDOM }
The state of not being imprisoned or enslaved.

When putting food at the heart of the matter, it's helpful to acknowledge and understand that there's a huge difference between choosing and enjoying your food from a place of freedom, acceptance and celebration, and choosing foods based on a deep fear of dying, ageing, and losing our energy and our ability to keep up with the demands of life.

Behind the shiny advertisements for superfoods and green smoothies is a belief that nothing will harm you if you eat these wonder products. Now I'm certainly not out to pan the chia seed or slander spirulina, but I want to point out that our quest for perfection – and the pride (and ultimately discouragement) that comes with it – can lead to a self-defeating 'immortality complex' approach to food.

THE IMMORTALITY MYTH

Put simply, it's time to lighten up a little, and return pure, unadulterated enjoyment to the food processor of life.

An 'immortality complex' is simply the mentality of an eater who is driven by the desire for an idealised state of health, and is also fleeing from the fear of sickness and death. You may be able to pick this Sherlock Holmes–type person out in a crowd. They'll be the one with a magnifying glass over an ingredients list or menu and who surveils their every twitch or symptom after indulging in a food they consider to be unhealthy or damaging.

The unfortunate truth of life is that no matter how hard we try to avoid illness and strive towards a state of physical perfection, we all have a time limit on our lives. We're all going to age, and even if you put significant effort and money into the perfect wonder diet and superfood regime, you could still encounter hurdles with your health, whether physical or emotional.

But even if you do achieve perfect health, there's no virtue in heading towards a life in the wellbeing 'bliss' zone if you're unconsciously projecting judgement, negativity and unhealthy standards on the people you influence, ensnaring them in a ripple effect of fear-driven food attitudes rather than the pure, simple, uncomplicated, untainted enjoyment of real food. Along with rediscovering balanced nutrition and simple pleasures, let's embrace a movement towards food freedom, one that makes food a foundational requirement and the cornerstone of living a supercharged life.

The time has come for us to be liberated and shake off burdensome agendas. Although physical immortality evades us, one of the best ways to embrace immortality is to have a positive impact on the planet and pass it on to future generations in a better state than we found it. Throughout this book I provide you with inspiring ways to do this.

Now I'm obviously not suggesting that we throw the baby out with the bathwater and foolishly mismanage our personal health, but I do believe we need to stop restricting certain ingredients we believe are a one-way ticket to the grave. Our biology of belief has just as great an impact on the way our food affects our body, as does the choice of that food itself. Let's vote for more freedom and balance in our lives, and feed our body according to its own needs.

PLEASURE

A feeling of happy satisfaction and enjoyment.

Pleasure is all around us, and the human condition is defined by our drive to seek it out. It's the little moments of wonder and happiness that make life beautiful and special: a striking piece of art, a song that brings up a beautiful memory, or the deep sense of contented joy that comes from being in the presence of loved ones. Yet ironically, in our cultural 'pursuit of happiness', we seem to have become numb to the everyday moments of squealish delight we should relish.

Through digital media, advertisements have made their way into every aspect and second of our day. And these images and messages are specifically designed to manipulate us into believing we have a multitude of problems that need urgent solutions or care. We seem to be working harder all the time, many of us in jobs we don't even like, to solve these manufactured 'problems' and to maintain a standard of living that's beyond our means and the capacity of our soul.

Because we're so busy, some of the 'solutions' that appeal to us are matters of convenience. And this is where I believe we've become completely cut off from the true pleasure of food. We live in an age where we're watching more cooking shows than ever before, yet we're spending less time in the kitchen. We're so gravely disconnected from our food that we've almost forgotten it's one of the keystones of life. Because we're a generation with constant access to the four seasons of produce from all corners of the earth, some of us may never understand the deep, sweet pleasure of that first spring pea after months and months of absence, or the taste of a luscious raspberry handpicked from the plant.

To reignite the pleasure of food, we must get back to a simple way of eating that's in synchronicity with the earth and its seasons, and create space in our own lives to be able to grow and gather our food, plan our meals, then cook and sit down at a table with enough time to truly savour their splendour.

Real food is our fuel, and in harnessing its true beauty, consuming mindfully and respecting the ideals of conservation, decentralisation, moderation and balance, we connect to the energy source that's vital for a supercharged life.

Food and the seven keystones of life

We're each here on earth to do great things, to honour the body we've been given, to nurture our soul, our mind, our immediate and wider family, and our community.

We've been designed with a body that can't function without eating, and we live on a planet that provides sustenance to our body beautifully if we work with nature's intelligence. Without food, we would cease to exist; it's the cornerstone of life.

Although it may seem like a mundane and repetitive ritual that's continually woven through our existence, eating is nevertheless a central practice in the life of every human. The way we interact with food, value it and set our behaviours around it has a subtle yet profound effect on our lives and our potential.

It can be useful in considering our approach to life to break it down into manageable parts. One of the easiest ways to do this is to consider the seven keystones of life (opposite). At number one and right at the centre is love, which is at the true heart of us all. But what magically weaves its way through our entire lives and brings every other keystone together is food.

Food reaches into our home and family, our friends and community, our career and passion, our spirituality, our finances, and also our health and longevity. Let's take a closer look at some of the ways food underpins and has the power to influence the seven keystones of life.

Home and family

In all cultures and throughout the ages, the kitchen has been regarded as the heart of the home and family. It's only in our fast-paced modern society that food has become an almost inconvenient necessity rather than something that draws people together. Mealtimes around the table at home, whether with flatmates, family, fur babies or just you, are where nourishment, both physical and emotional, begins. Embracing self-leadership, and leadership in your home when it comes to the quality of the food you prepare, has an impact on you and your household's health and wellbeing that radiates out into the world. Food is the very heart of the home.

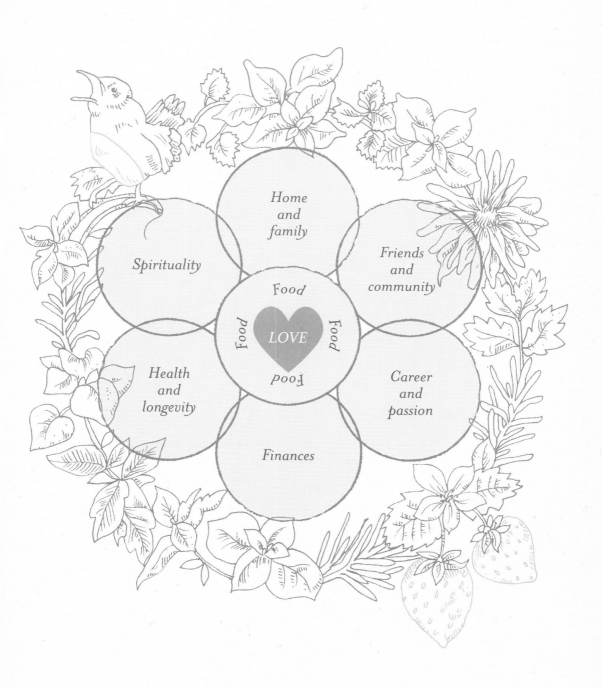

Friends and community

The simple act of sharing a meal is the cement that holds our relationships and community together. Celebrations of life and even death are often centred around food and drinks. Socialisation in our culture is almost always connected to drinks, whether it's coffee in a café or a wine with friends after work. Cooking meals is a practical way of showing love, care and support to friends in need. At every level, food binds communities together and strengthens friendships and a sense of belonging. Food is connection, it brings us together.

Career and passion

Food costs money, and our need to source a living drives us into the workplace. Isn't it interesting to think that, fundamentally, we go to work so we can eat three meals a day? On the other hand, our personal growth, productivity and capacity to be creative and effective in our career are largely determined by the state of our health – which is directly linked to the lifestyle we lead and the types of food we use to fuel our body. This means that when we invest in quality healthy food, we're more likely to thrive in our careers and have the energy to live a life aligned to our true purpose and passion. Food is our life force, our *prana*.

Finances

We have a responsibility to vote for the kind of world we live in through our wallets and finances. Every purchase we make has a backstory. The food we invest in can either be depleting the earth's soil of nutrients, pushing farmers into debt and hardship, and propagating unethical work practices; or it can be working with the intelligence of nature and the seasons, providing a fair income for workers, and contributing to a healthier society at large. Food as an investment, with smart meal planning and budgeting, can also act as a beautiful source of fulfilment in our lives. Food is our future.

Health and longevity

It's no secret that food is directly linked to our personal health and the health of our population. The cost of obesity and other food-related illnesses is rising and placing an increasing burden on society. Yet a healthy lifestyle that favours an abundance of seasonal real foods will cut down the costs of visits to the doctor and prescription drugs to treat the symptoms of underlying health issues. The food we choose to eat can be the key to a long life, and the health benefits of good food can help us experience and enjoy life fully, right into old age. Food is our lifeline.

Spirituality

The way nature provides the plants and animals we eat with medicinal and nourishing properties that allow our bodies to function and thrive is a divine source of wonderment in and of itself. The spiritual beliefs of many traditional hunter-gatherer societies include a deep sense of awe for the provisions of nature. It's as if the earth has a mind of its own, and provides and blesses the bodies and needs of its people.

The respect that comes with a spiritual connection to the earth's provision of food is a far cry from the West's vast disconnect from the death and sacrifice of the animal that sits in a packet on the supermarket shelf. Having a spiritual practice is a beautiful way to reframe your respect and gratitude for the earth and the food it provides. Food is our belief system.

Love

Hospitality is a language of the heart and has always existed as a way to serve and show love to those most important to us. The desire to nourish others is an in-built instinct. Food also has the power to set the mood for romance, with aphrodisiac foods like oysters a way to ignite the flames of sexuality and passion. Sitting down to a candlelit meal is a special way to show how much you value someone you love, and provides opportunity for deep conversation that cuts through surface-level banter and moves right through to the heart, improving your soul connection and forging a deeper sense of unity. Food is love.

The beauty of your personal food culture

Food plays a key role in the story of our life. The way we interact with it will have consequences for us personally – physically, socially, culturally, spiritually and emotionally. Likewise, the way we make choices about food (or interact with it passively) will have wider consequences for the world around us.

Have you ever thought about the potential influence you can have on yourself, those around you and the world you live in just through the way you interact culturally with food? A food culture is simply how an individual or a group of people interacts with and thinks about food. This can be the result of a multitude of factors, ranging from family and national heritage to the media, language, social trends, tradition, ethics, spirituality and more.

Traditionally, food cultures have been predominantly passed down by mothers, who perpetuated the food wisdom and knowledge of cooking they inherited from their own mothers and grandmothers. A lot has changed in our modern society to break this traditional chain of transmitted food cultures. Today, many mothers are busy in the workforce, which is a wonderful thing. It does make it hard, however, for either partner to play a primary role as nourishing parent. While some families are still managing to maintain a traditional food culture, many children are being raised according to the nutritional standards of their schools and childcare centres, the dictates of the media, and the values of convenience over tradition.

The beauty of culture is that it can be created intentionally. Though it might seem like something that just forms on its own and influences your life from the outside, culture can be engineered. You have the power to create and nurture culture in your sphere of influence, whether that's your personal life, household, peer group or workplace. This is true leadership, and it lies at the heart of living a supercharged life.

CREATING YOUR OWN FOOD CULTURE

The first step is to figure out your values concerning food. You can probably articulate your value system cogently, but can you do the same when it comes to food? Our food values can stem from a range of factors, as you're about to see. So grab a pen and paper, and get ready to brainstorm.

Heritage

Family and heritage often play a key role in food values. This is often closely linked with nationality or your cultural identity and the foods you may have grown up with. Are there recipes, beliefs and memories concerning food that you wish to pass down to your children or loved ones? Almost everyone will have a series of food memories that define who they are, whether it's their Italian nonna teaching them how to make pasta, or their father taking them on a camping trip and cooking a special recipe over an open fire.

Think about the recipes, memories and values around food that have come from your own heritage. Which ones do you want to carry through into your own food culture?

Attitudes

We all have attitudes and beliefs regarding food, largely as a result of the thinking we were brought up with, but also developed from the attitudes of the society and culture we live in.

Many of these attitudes can be damaging. The media, for example, often generates fear and confusion about food through marketing, news stories and diet fads. It's important not to allow our values to be hijacked and driven by these wishy-washy attitudes to food, which arise more from agenda-driven fear-mongering than common sense. Where have your food beliefs been formed?

Your parents may have shown you a love of nature and the blessing of food and its preparation; or they may have seen cooking as a burdensome chore, creating an attitude of negativity around food. Write down some of your own negative attitudes to food and cooking that you now wish to discard, and replace them with positive ones that will help you create a new culture of appreciation, gratitude and joy for food and cooking.

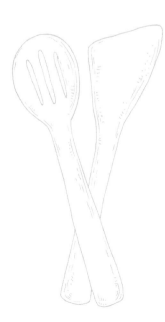

Language

What words do you use to describe food? Are they negative or positive? You may have been brought up with a way of talking about food that doesn't place value on it or on cooking. You may not even realise the complaining words that can come out of your mouth when faced with the task of cooking or eating a meal that doesn't satisfy your expectations. The words you use to describe food can create a culture either of discontent, negativity and entitlement, or of appreciation, gratitude and privilege. Think deeply about the words you choose to describe food. Food is special!

Spirituality

Do you follow a particular religion or spiritual practice? Many religions and world views have corresponding cultural practices that range from the rejection of certain foods on moral grounds to fasting, rituals and celebratory recipes, as well as the practice of giving thanks before meals. Beliefs concerning creation and the character of your god or gods will also impact on your moral interaction with food. What are your spiritual beliefs and how can they be incorporated into your personal food culture?

Social values

Do you value food for its ability to create community? Do you value hospitality? These are important questions if you want to have a social impact on those around you. One of your food culture values might be, for example, that you always sit down to meals in your home, and that the table is a place of enjoyment and nourishment but also a chance to connect and deepen relationships. You might also have standards and practices about the way you entertain people who come over for dinner, and see food as an opportunity to reveal your value for others and express generosity. Think about the practicalities of what that looks like for you and jot them down.

Morals, ethics and political views

This keystone is largely linked to the spiritual and to your own personal world view. Consider the morals and ethical standards you wish to express through your food culture. You might wish to resist conventional food marketing, instead holding to a philosophy of real and traditional food.

Or you might practise vegetarianism due to your moral beliefs about the treatment of animals. Or you might instead wish to purchase only organic, grass-fed, free-range meats and other animal products.

On a philosophical level, I encourage you to embrace an approach termed 'metamodernism'. It means engaging not only in dialogue but in collaboration, and is a lens for thinking about the self, language, culture and meaning in an open, supportive and engaged way. Other people's food cultures and food choices – such as veganism or the paleo diet – might be very different from our own. But rather than being diametrically opposed to those positions, metamodernism encourages us to recognise both sides and consciously try to join our efforts and perspectives with those of others. This means that no matter how different other people's viewpoints and subjectivities might be from ours, we can still find common ground with them and create a sense of collaboration rather than conflict.

On a political level, you might like to avoid supermarkets and choose to support local farmers, co-ops, farmers' markets and community-based agriculture that will boost your local economy. Fair-trade products may be important to you, and you might wish to know the story of your food before investing in it. The metamodern approach allows you to view your own food culture and choices with both sincerity and awareness, and to alternate with self-awareness between positions that offer what works for you.

Living a supercharged life begins with you considering your food culture and what it means to you, and applying those values and principles within your life in a way that doesn't judge people who choose to live otherwise.

Once you explore and understand how to express your food culture in your own life, you'll be on your way to establishing your supercharged kitchen. As you read through this book, you can start setting the scene and pulling together your fundamental equipment needs, then learn how to build your meals by cultivating flavour and giving it prominence.

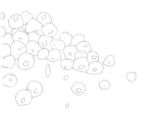

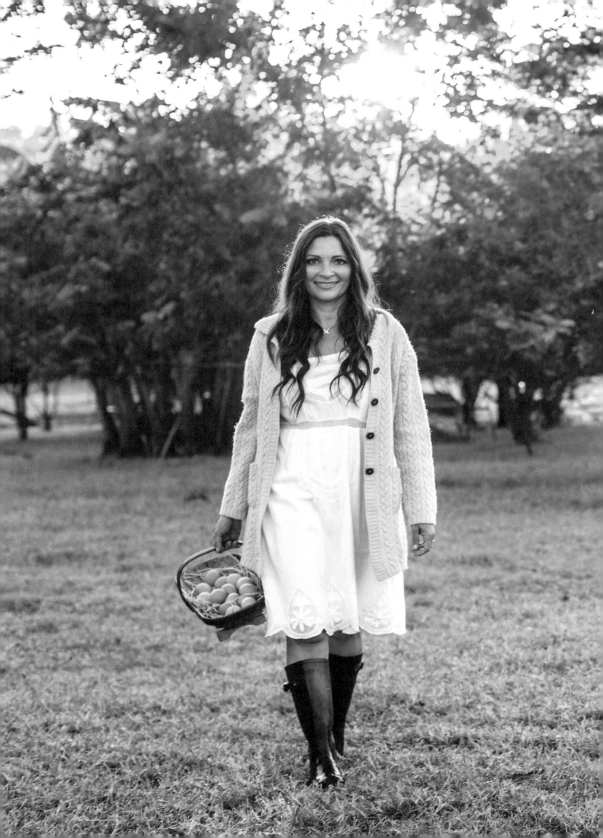

PART·ONE

eat

{ *PAGES* 23 — 135 }

Outfitting an enduring kitchen

The kitchen is the heart of the home, but if you're new to home cooking, fear not – you don't have to be an expert or spend a bajillion dollars setting up a supercharged kitchen. All you're trying to achieve is a way to cook and feed yourself, family and friends that optimises the amount of time and money spent, and allows food to become the heart of your home.

You can thrive on the simplest and most natural meals, made with the minimum of fuss and based on fresh vegetables and fruit, nuts, meats, simple salads and desserts. It's sometimes fun, however, to mix up your meals so you don't get bored. You want to be able to create situations where you can derive pleasure and fulfilment from your food as well as nourishment.

The first step towards an enduring supercharged kitchen is to ensure you have at your disposal the food preparation options you need. The following is a list of the kitchen equipment I use most when creating my dishes at home. Depending on your lifestyle and financial position, you may not require them all – just pick and choose what will work for you. When it comes to outfitting, aim for a minimalist kitchen where less is more.

Spiraliser
The spiraliser is an inexpensive tool that can add variety to your meals, turning basic vegetable into oodles of noodles. Don't think of these as just for the carb-conscious or healthy chefs; everyone from home cooks to kids is spiralising and eating up their vegetables in the process. Pick a firm peeled or unpeeled vegie – zucchinis and carrots work well – and watch as it's transformed into a pile of extra-long, gently curled noodles or ribbons you can enjoy as a fun dish.

High-speed blender
A high-speed blender will perhaps be one of the more expensive items you invest in, but this one sturdy and versatile central piece of kitchen equipment is worth every penny. High-speed blenders can perform certain tasks that 'regular' blenders can't, such as making nut butters and milks, whipping up instant 'ice creams', grinding coffee beans, and

creating extremely smooth drinks. It's time to say goodbye to 'sip and chew' green smoothies. If you gravitate towards eating raw food, a high-speed blender will enable you to extract all the fibre and juice from your fresh produce (there's no pulp residue), which means better value when it comes to ingredient budgeting and less waste. You'll notice that high-speed blenders vary dramatically in price. Rather than pay a premium for a brand name, I'd recommend purchasing a blender with a good warranty, as you want it to be a long-lasting investment.

Food processor

A food processor is your ally when it comes to reducing your kitchen preparation work. I use mine for a number of tasks, from shredding and chopping vegetables to creating pesto sauces and bliss balls, blending sauces and salsas, making crusts and doughs, and chopping nuts and grinding them into flours. My advice would be to choose a model that's easy to clean and has a strong processing speed. If you're tossing up whether to invest in a high-speed blender or food processor, they both have their distinct advantages, so look at what your kitchen needs and what you do most, then work back from there.

Dehydrator

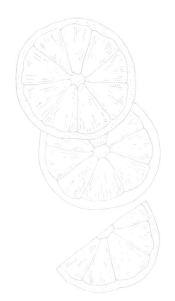

While definitely not an essential item – an oven on low heat can essentially perform the same function – a dehydrator is a worthwhile investment if you intend to create ready-to-go foods such as crackers, biscuits, vegetable and fruit straps, and vegetable chips. It can also help you cut down on food wastage by drying herbs and fruits for later use.

Dehydrated food will keep for much longer, so you can dehydrate an assembly line of produce over the weekend when you have some spare time. Dehydrating typically takes between four and 12 hours depending on the kind of ingredients you're using. I store my dehydrated foods in airtight jars and containers. Home food dehydrators fall into two categories: those with stackable trays, and those consisting of a rigid box with removable shelves. Size is a factor; most fit on a benchtop, but larger models are free-standing and require more space.

Cast-iron pans

These may seem a bit on the old-fashioned side, but they're a must in a supercharged kitchen: they conduct heat beautifully, dance from stovetop to oven with no issues, and last for decades. The sheen on cast-iron cookware renders it virtually non-stick, allowing you to use less oil in your dishes.

Roasting tins

Although a variety of tins may be suitable for roasting, roasting tins are particularly useful for cooking large pieces of meat to feed the whole family. The bottoms and sides of these tins will radiate and intensify an oven's heat, browning the outside of your food quickly while keeping the inside moist. The pan itself will catch and brown any cooking liquids for later use in a gravy or marinade. Enamelled cast-iron roasters are the best as they provide steady, even heat. Look for one that's heavily enamelled, as thin coatings can chip or crack and have a shorter lifespan.

Chargrill pans and woks

Chargrill pans and woks, preferably enamelled cast-iron versions, are fantastic when preparing Asian-style dishes. I like to get the most out of mine by using them to reheat food – they yield a more delicious result than a microwave.

Wooden spoons and spatulas

Wooden spoons are the ideal mixing tool. They're strong, won't scratch the finish of your cookware, are insulated (and thus won't cause sudden temperature changes in your food), have a high heat tolerance and are eco-friendly. Avoid plastics and silicone. Although they're more flexible, it's best to stay away from them, largely for environmental reasons but also for health reasons, especially around hot liquids. I'd suggest using metal spatulas and slotted spoons, metal-tipped tongs and wooden spoons. But don't throw out perfectly serviceable cookware unless you think it poses a genuine health risk. It's greener to keep old utensils than replace them with new ones.

Top three knives

The only three knives you really need in your kitchen are a 20 cm (8 inch) chef's knife for chopping vegies and herbs, slicing meat and whacking hard shells such as coconuts; a sharp paring knife for peeling fruit and vegies; and a bread knife for slicing bread and tomatoes, and levelling cakes and bakes.

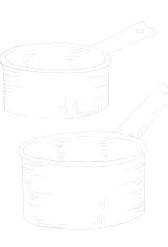

Mixing bowls and measuring cups and spoons

With the planet in mind, choose wooden, bamboo or metal vessels rather than plastic ones. These will make your recipe-creation experience much easier and will also last much longer.

Sieves, strainers and colanders

Sieves are great for creating ultra-light baked goods – simply sift any flours before mixing them in. With colanders, choose metal rather than plastic. I have a large colander for straining larger items such as steamed vegies and pastas, and a finer-meshed strainer for smaller items such as rice.

Scales

A good set of kitchen scales will make following recipes much easier. We've all been guilty of over- or underestimating the weight of our meats, only to burn them to a crisp or serve them half-raw!

Citrus juicer

You may be able to get away without one, but the extra juice you'll be able to extract from your citrus fruits will definitely make up for the investment, and will mean less wastage. You might find that your food processor has an attachment for this.

Grater

When choosing a grater, be sure to select one that's firm, with a strong steady base, so that it won't slide as you grate your food. Most food processors have a grating function and, depending on the intended use of the grated food, the job it does might be adequate for your needs.

Now you're armed with all the necessary ideas for utensils, your only challenge will be choosing which delicious meal to prepare first. But before you start deciding which recipes you want to try, make sure you read on. I want to demystify any misconceptions you may have about true flavour, and explain the art of flavour cultivation.

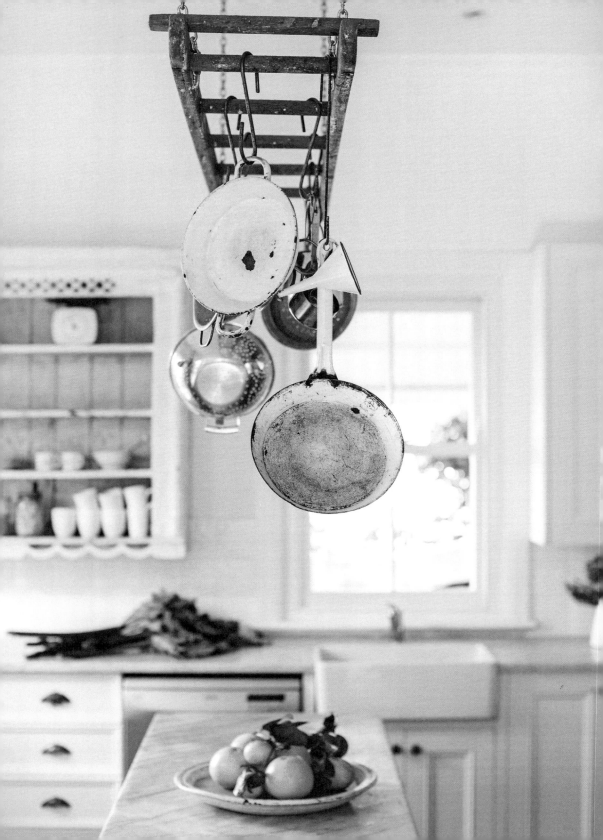

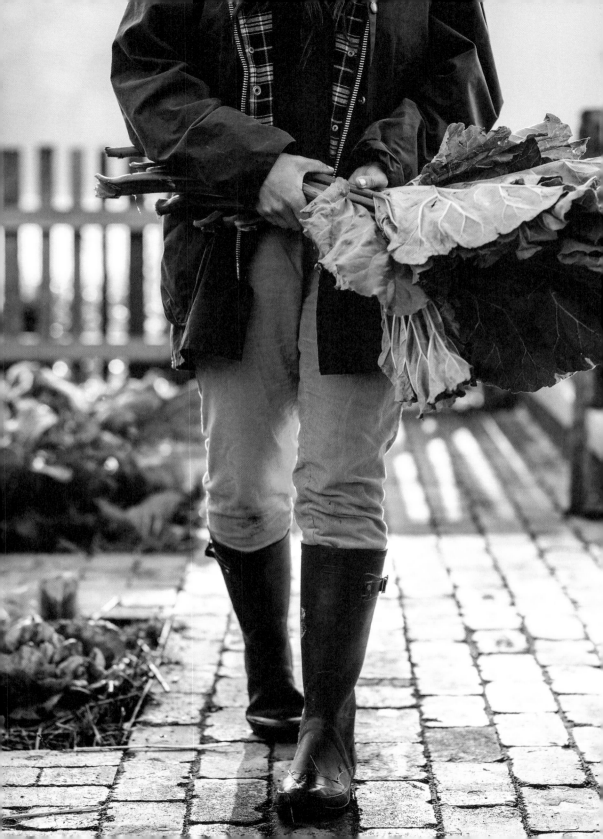

Cultivating flavour

{ FLAVOUR }
The indication of the essential character of something.

True flavour is created at the hands of a cook – a human, not a machine or a production line. It's lovingly selected from real, raw ingredients from Mother Earth. It's the alchemy of these personally chosen ingredients, drawn together with love and skill, that produces genuine character in a dish.

As children, we're first introduced to different flavours by the foods our parents feed us. From then on, as we become more self-sufficient and begin eating more independently, going to friends' houses and trying different cultural cuisines, we learn and accumulate knowledge of what tastes good to us through a lifelong process of trial and error.

Peanut butter and jam (jelly), mint and chocolate, salt and vinegar: these food pairings are all enjoyed by most of us, regardless of our age, economic background or gender. But have you ever stopped to think why this is?

Each food has its own 'flavour profile', which is a breakdown of how it tastes. These profiles can be formulated using just a handful of universal flavour elements, such as sweet, salty, bitter, sour and the Japanese favourite called 'umami' or savoury. Spicy and fatty can also be included here. In Ayurvedic philosophies, the sense of taste is a natural roadmap directing us towards good nutrition and characterised by six individual tastes: sweet, sour, salty, bitter, astringent and pungent (I cover these in my Ayurvedic cookbook *Eat Right for Your Shape*).

Texture also plays an important role in food, as it allows certain ingredients to enhance the satisfying flavour of others. Just think how much better crunchy croutons taste when they're tossed in creamy soups or served over crisp salads rather than eaten as a stand-alone snack. Bitter and salty are the only flavour elements that actually enhance the flavours of other ingredients, while the other elements act more to complement one another.

Food pairing in molecular gastronomy is based on the principle that foods combine well with one another when they share key flavour components. All foods contain flavour compounds. A compound called isoamyl acetate, for example, is what gives bananas and pears their distinct aromas.

FLAVOUR PAIRING

Flavour pairing is simply combining foods that have the same flavour compounds. Over the past ten years there have been some impressive findings in the study of human taste biochemistry. Chefs implement this notion of molecular gastronomy in preparing their dishes, often with unique yet tantalising results – my own Roasted Fig, Walnut and Goat's Cheese Salad (page 50) comes to mind here. Combining certain foods can also increase their nutritional value, helping your body absorb and utilise the benefits of each separate ingredient more effectively. It seems the whole really is greater than the sum of its parts.

It just so happens that our mouths like to maintain a careful balance between flavours. For example, if a food is too bitter, we look for something sweet to counterbalance it. If a food is too salty, we look for something with a higher water content and bland flavour to balance it out. The concept of creating perfect flavour pairings is employed by chefs, sommeliers, food technologists and even perfumers.

We all know couples who just seem to complement each other perfectly. One is a talker, the other is shy; one is daring, the other conservative; one is a hot mess, the other a neat freak. The same principle of power couples can be applied to food.

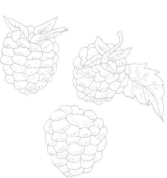

It's quite incredible what our palates are capable of appreciating, and by employing a few simple molecular gastronomy principles, you too can create simple, healthy, chef-inspired meals all in the comfort of your own home. On the following pages are six of the most common food pairings that combine effortlessly – think of it as a handy guide to perfect partners. Some of these you might have heard of, others may seem a little out of the ordinary (like my Sea Salt, Fresh Raspberry and Slivered Almond Chocolate, page 56). Be inspired to experiment a little with different ingredients and flavours, and reap the rewards by tantalising your tastebuds.

Sweet and sour

Think of sour gummy bears. The concept of sweet and sour is one that Asian cuisines frequently employ, particularly in their sauces and soups. Try creating your own sweet and sour snacks by drizzling apple cider vinegar over strawberries, or squeezing lime juice over ripe pineapple. The sweetness of fruit helps counter the bitterness and acidity of the vinegar and lime juice, which, if consumed by themselves, have a tendency to make us pull all sorts of unflattering faces.

Salt and fatty

This is a principle employed all too often by major fast-food chains. Think French fries, fried chicken and sky-high beef burgers. In my supercharged kitchen I simply roast some sweet potatoes in a little coconut oil, season them with Himalayan salt and spice – I particularly love cumin and paprika – and bake at low heat until crispy. Or you could try my Cumin-spiced Lotus Root Chips (page 120).

Sweet and fatty

Chocolate croissants, French toast, French fries dipped in soft serve – does this sound familiar? Combining the luxurious, creamy texture of fatty foods with sweet flavours sends our tastebuds straight to heaven and puts our pleasure pathways on high alert. Whatever combination of ingredients you put together, breakfast or dessert are fun places to begin. Why not try my delicious Raw Chocolate Tart with Berry Sauce (page 286) or create a mixed berry and coconut milk smoothie – just whiz in a high-speed blender and bombs away.

Sweet and spicy

Chilli chocolate is just one example of a sweet and spicy flavour combination. A simple snack that exploits this unique pairing and takes only a few minutes to create is sweet chilli walnuts. Simply coat some walnuts in rice malt syrup or another sticky sweetener of choice, season with chilli, remembering not to go overboard, and roast at low heat until they turn golden brown and crunchy. These make great movie snacks for those long streaming nights.

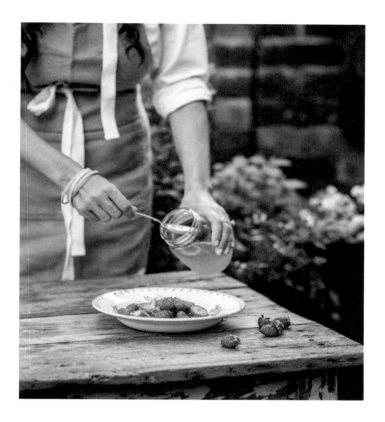

Sweet and salty

You often see this pairing in delicatessens. Cheese platters with dried fruits and prosciutto wrapped around rockmelon are two delicious examples. I tend to apply this principle often in my salads, such as my lazy-person's salad containing some fresh greens, lemon juice, tomatoes, olives and watermelon. Dress this combo with a little extra virgin olive oil and Himalayan salt, and be transported to flavour paradise.

Sweet and savoury

Dessert recipes make great use of this combination. Think zucchini muffins or my Layered Salted Caramel Peanut Fudge (page 295). If you get the outfitting of your supercharged kitchen sorted, you can participate in this magic in the comfort of your own home. Once mastered, you'll find it one of the greatest joys of cooking.

Rather than relying on pre-made flavour mixes and seasonings, the first step to imparting flavour to your meals is stocking up on the right single ingredients that can be brought together in hundreds of unique combinations to make unparalleled dishes.

MAKING A GOOD MARINADE

I love that cooking has a dual benefit. It allows us to nourish and fulfil our body through the choice of supercharged ingredients, but it can also tantalise the heck out of our tastebuds with crafty combinations of flavours! Understanding how to combine and balance flavours, as well as strengthening flavour through marinating, will help you really nail your foodie creations.

Marinating is an age-old process and the easiest way to intensify the flavour of food before cooking with a few basic ingredients. Marinades can be pastes, liquids or dry rubs, and they are mainly used for meats, but can also be used for vegies. Marinating tougher cuts of meat is best done overnight in the fridge. Fish, chicken breasts and tender cuts of beef or lamb fillet are better marinated for a shorter time – a couple of hours, say.

Marinades will typically include three basic components:

1 OILS: The oil content prevents the meat drying out and really binds together and locks in the flavour. The best oils for marinating include olive and sesame oil. Coconut oil, however, solidifies in the fridge, inhibiting the flavours from moving freely and permeating the meat.

2 ACIDS: These unravel the proteins in the meat, making it beautifully tender and softening the surface to allow the flavours to permeate. My favourite acids are apple cider vinegar, balsamic vinegar, brown rice vinegar, pomegranate juice, preservative-free organic wine, citrus juice, yoghurt, and coconut milk combined with lemon or lime juice (a great dairy-free buttermilk substitute).

3 SEASONINGS: These include dried and fresh herbs and spices (see pages 58–65), sea salt, pepper, coconut sugar, citrus zest, tamari, honey, rice malt syrup, tamarind and other flavour-balancing ingredients you can use to achieve the kind of vibe you're after. Sugars will enhance browning and caramelisation of your meat, while salty components will enhance the natural glutamates and savoury flavours.

A good basic marinade recipe includes one part acid, one part oil, and one to two parts seasoning, balancing salty and sweet with your chosen herbs and spices. Use enough to coat the quantity of meat or vegetables, and leave them covered in the fridge for the appropriate time until cooking.

For dry spice rubs, choose flavours in the ratio of four parts sea salt to three parts sugar (coconut sugar works well) and three parts spices. Rubs are best used for meats rather than fish. Rub all over the nooks and crannies of your meat, wrap in plastic wrap and leave up to 72 hours if need be. Spice rubs are best used on meat to be grilled or oven-roasted.

FLAVOUR COMBINATIONS

Take these complementary flavours into account when pairing ingredients in your kitchen creations

- **WHITE FISH:** *apple cider vinegar, butter, capers, chilli with tamari and ginger, coconut, coriander (cilantro), dill, fennel, lemon, lime, olives and tomato, parsley, saffron, star anise, thyme, white wine*
- **OILY FISH:** *almonds, asparagus, avocado, beetroot, chilli, cumin, dill, garlic, ginger, lemon, lime*
- **LAMB:** *apricots, cardamom, cinnamon, coriander, cumin, ginger, lemon and garlic, onion, peas and mint, pine nuts, rosemary, sweet potato, thyme, yoghurt*
- **BEEF:** *bay leaf, broccoli, celery and carrot, chilli, cloves, ginger, lime and coriander, mushrooms, olives, onions, orange zest, parsley, red wine*
- **CHICKEN:** *almonds, avocado, basil, cashews, celery, chilli, coconut, garlic, lemon, lime, mushrooms, saffron, sage, thyme*

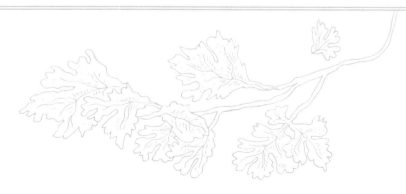

NINE WINNING FLAVOUR COMBOS

When looking to bolster your energy with flavour-enriching combinations, here are nine playful ways to marry ingredients, obtain the flavour you desire and boost your overall health.

1 **Beans, tomatoes, berries and capsicums (peppers)**
Increase your absorption of non-haem iron by consuming foods such as beans in combination with a source of vitamin C, such as oranges, tomatoes, berries and capsicums.

2 **Green tea, mint and lemon, lime or grapefruit juice**
Consumed together, green tea, mint and citrus juice will help you absorb significantly more antioxidants. Adding a splash of citrus juice to green tea reduces the breakdown of its catechins (a type of antioxidant) in your digestive system. It's also a refreshing drink to have first thing in the morning before you tuck in to breakfast.

3 **Fatty fish, garlic, ginger, broccoli and basil**
This combination, often employed in Greek cuisine and several Asian cultures, strikes the perfect balance between rich and mild flavours. Heart-healthy antioxidants found in foods such as garlic, ginger and broccoli may be responsible for improved absorption of omega-3 fats.

4 **Yoghurt, rice malt syrup and bananas**
This combination makes the perfect post-workout snack, as consuming these foods together after exercise may aid muscle recovery. The combination of the carbohydrates (from the bananas and rice malt syrup) with the protein (found in dairy foods) enhances the insulin response, helping the body to soak up nutrients. Children are also enamoured of this ultimate calming combo.

TRY THIS: Blend 125 ml (4 fl oz/½ cup) of your favourite plant-based milk, 130 g (4½ oz/½ cup) organic unsweetened yoghurt, 1 medium banana (use a frozen banana for a thicker consistency if you have a high-speed blender) and 1 tablespoon rice malt syrup or raw honey. Add pinches of ground cinnamon, nutmeg and ginger (optional) to create a creamy, delicious smoothie.

---

5   Apples, berries, walnuts, coconut, cinnamon
    and cloves
    If apples and berries could speak, they'd say to each other
    'You complete me!' The antioxidant ellagic acid (found in
    pomegranates, walnuts, cranberries and raspberries) enhances
    the potency of the antioxidant quercetin (found in grapes,
    onion, buckwheat and apples).

6   Green leafy vegetables, raw salad greens, avocado,
    nuts, seeds, plant-based oils and tomatoes
    To derive the full range of benefits from your vegies, avoid
    fat-free dressings and opt for real and healthy fats such
    as olive oil, diced avocado, nuts and seeds. Fat-soluble
    antioxidants like those found in tomatoes and leafy greens
    are better absorbed and easier to digest when combined
    with some healthy fat.

7   Seafood, rice, salt and fermented vegies
    The saltiness of these foods balances the subtle and mild
    flavours of steamed rice and fish. No wonder sushi and soy
    sauce is such a popular lunchtime option. The probiotics in
    fermented foods such as sauerkraut, kimchi, soy and tamari aid
    digestion of the proteins and carbohydrates in fish and rice.

8   Oily fish, eggs, bread, avocado, lettuce, salt
    and pepper
    There's something about an egg-mayo sandwich that sends
    most people's pleasure receptors into a flutter. The creaminess
    of the mayonnaise perfectly balances the richness of the
    eggs and the low notes of the bread. Seasoning with salt and
    pepper gives distinct flavour to what would otherwise be
    a slightly ho-hum sandwich.

9   Red meat, rice malt syrup, tamari, sage
    and rosemary
    Sweet and savoury at its best – the sweetness of rice malt
    syrup complements the saltiness of the tamari and enhances
    the buttery texture of the fat from the red meat. It's no wonder
    that herb-infused, sweetly glazed roast meat dishes have been
    a family dinner staple for centuries.

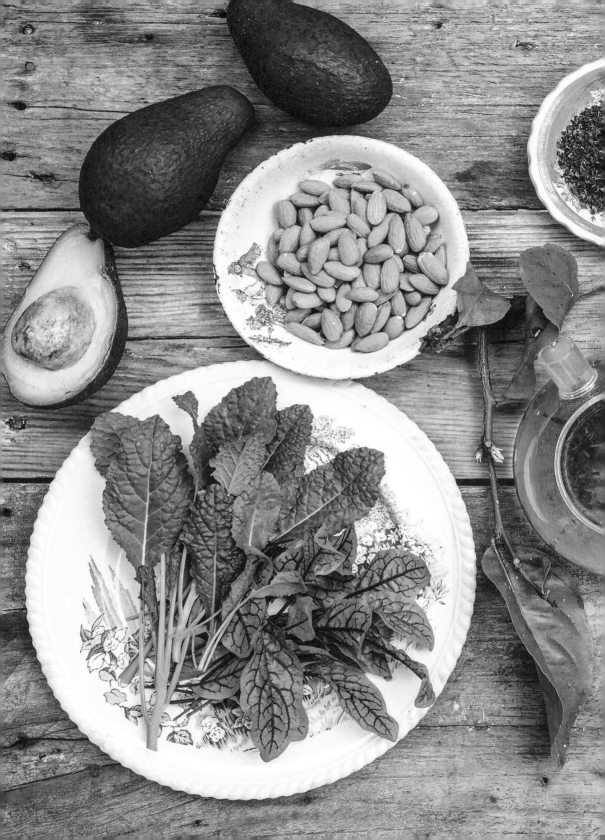

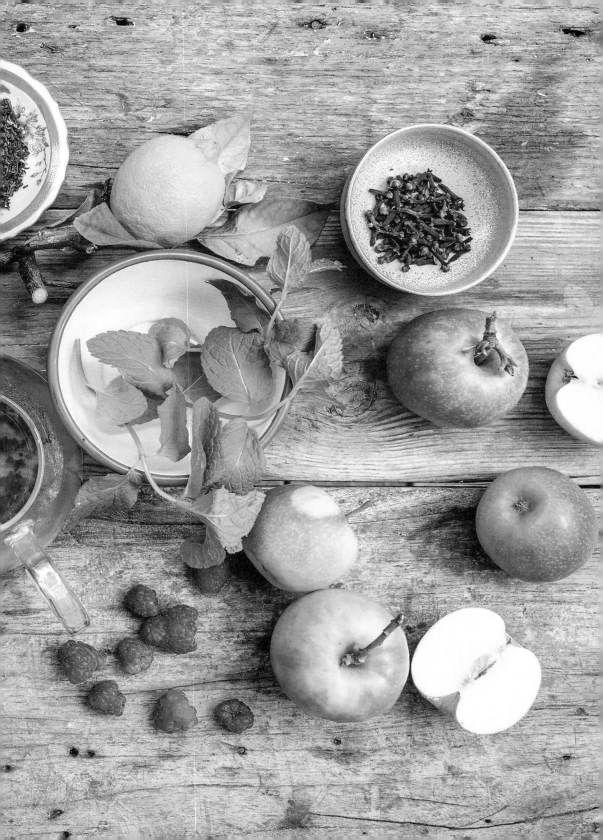

PERFECT FOOD PAIRINGS

INGREDIENTS	PROTEIN FOODS	HERBS	RECIPE IDEAS
Artichokes, chilli, lentils, mushrooms, nuts, potatoes, tomatoes	Beef, chicken, tuna	Bay leaf, oregano, thyme	Stocks, soups, bolognese sauces, poached seafood, casseroles, my Supercharged Shakshuka (page 68) with tuna
Cauliflower, garlic, mushrooms, onion, potatoes, spinach, tomatoes	Eggs, beef, turkey	Rosemary, thyme, sage	Roast meats, frittatas
Cabbage, carrots, cucumber, garlic, ginger, mustard, onion, pepper, yoghurt	Fish, chicken, eggs	Basil, dill, chives, fennel	Pickles, stews, tzatziki, my Chermoula Prawn and Shaved Fennel Salad (page 158)

TRY THIS: For a healthy, bone-building sandwich alternative, make an egg, avocado, dill and salad filling on slices of spelt or wholegrain bread. If eggs aren't your thing, substitute an oily fish such as salmon. Season with Himalayan salt and freshly ground black pepper.

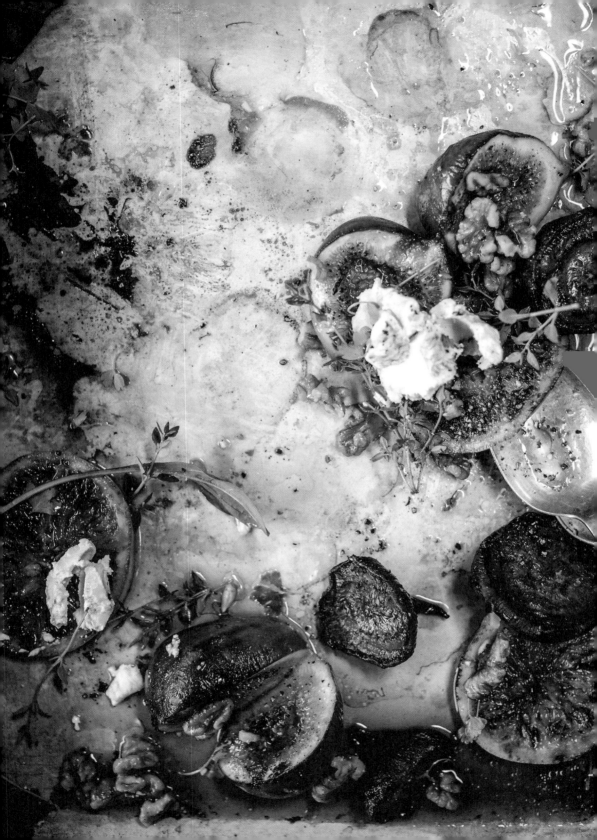

When I'm in the kitchen and want to enhance or balance particular flavours, I whip out a few of my supercharged mainstay ingredients to help me achieve equilibrium for the tastebuds. I prefer to add small quantities and taste-test as I go.

FINDING BALANCE

Certain flavours balance others by counteracting or offsetting them to achieve harmony on the palate. For example, if you're cooking and you've accidently dropped too much spice into the pan, you can bring a sweet ingredient into play to balance and neutralise the heat. If you intend to enhance or amplify a sweet flavour, try adding a touch of saltiness. Salted caramel chocolate, come at me!

Try the gentle art of balancing by employing these tastes, and when in doubt, like everything in life, listen to your gut and trust your instincts.

- SOURNESS/ACIDITY can brighten a dish and give it vivacity, like lime on avocado. I favour lemon juice, lime juice, apple cider vinegar and brown rice vinegar.
- SWEETNESS can be used to balance sourness, bitterness and spiciness. Try rice malt syrup, maple syrup, raw honey, mirin and stevia drops or powder.
- SALTINESS brings out the flavours and aromas of other ingredients in a dish, and helps to reduce bitterness. I reach for wheat-free tamari, coconut aminos, and Celtic sea salt or Himalayan salt.
- BITTERNESS can be used to balance a dish that's too sweet, rich and heavy. Ingredients that can help include citrus peel, raw cacao powder and dandelion root.

For flavouring a dish, I gravitate towards green, grassy, herby flavours in the form of fresh parsley, coriander (cilantro), sage, dill, oregano, rosemary and thyme. My herb garden gets quite a workout most days. Grounding flavours can be achieved with garlic, onions, shallots and leeks.

If you've attempted the balancing acts above and your creation still seems lacklustre, why not try adding a umami-rich ingredient? I chop up an anchovy to give my bolognese a boost, wheat-free tamari is wonderful in soups, slow-cooking and stir-fries (try the Cauliflower Fried Rice, page 181), or add a hint of parmesan or nutritional yeast flakes, as in my Oven-baked Broccoli and Cauliflower Steaks (page 126).

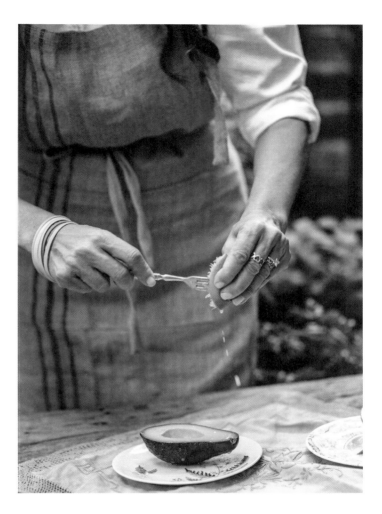

Think of your dish as creating a piece of music – you might start with the bass and then add layers as you go. It's the same in cooking, where we categorise flavours as notes from which we can create a symphony. Low notes are flavours that linger and set the groundwork for other flavours; they're usually earthy and umami. Mid-notes such as chicken and cauliflower are subtle and understated, and don't tend to stick around as long as the others. High notes are the effervescent show ponies that sparkle and dance around your tastebuds, such as lime or lemon, or chilli or paprika.

Enjoy experimenting in your supercharged kitchen, and remember the best recipes are usually simple, heartfelt and made with love.

Minted mango tropical crush

{ *SERVES* 2 }

1 mango, peeled and sliced

250 ml (9 fl oz/1 cup) coconut
  milk

250 ml (9 fl oz/1 cup) coconut
  water

juice of 1 lime

90 g (3¼ oz/2 cups) baby
  English spinach leaves

1 tablespoon nut butter

handful mint leaves, plus extra
  to serve

handful ice cubes

coconut flakes, to serve
  (optional)

Whiz all the ingredients except the coconut
flakes in a high-speed blender or food
processor until combined. Serve topped with
a sprig of extra mint and some coconut flakes,
if using.

White chocolate chai

{ *SERVES* 2 }

When you're craving a comforting dessert but don't want anything heavy, give
this super-cosy hot drink a try. It will wrap its arms around you, and make you
feel loved and supported. Cacao butter is the real superstar here, bringing
forth a pure and genuine white chocolate flavour.

55 g (2 oz/¼ cup) grated cacao
  butter

500 ml (17 fl oz/2 cups) coconut
  milk

generous pinch of ground
  ginger

generous pinch of ground
  cinnamon, plus extra to serve

generous pinch of freshly
  grated nutmeg

3 cardamom pods

2 cloves

Melt the cacao butter in a small saucepan over
low heat, stirring occasionally, then add the
coconut milk. Add the remaining ingredients,
increase the heat to medium and gently bring
to the boil, then reduce the heat to low and
allow the flavours to infuse for 5 minutes.
Strain and serve in favourite mugs with extra
cinnamon sprinkled on top (see tip).

SUPERCHARGED TIP
If you like your chai sweeter, add honey.

Kale and strawberry smoothie bowl

{ *SERVES* 2 }

Smoothie bowls are thick and creamy smoothies you can eat for breakfast, topped with delicious add-ons. You can make them the night before and refrigerate if your mornings fly by in a hurry.

½ ripe avocado, peeled

2 frozen bananas

250 g (9 oz) fresh or frozen strawberries

2 large handfuls baby English spinach leaves

2 kale leaves, spines removed

375 ml (13 fl oz/1½ cups) coconut or almond milk, plus extra as needed

1 tablespoon flaxseed meal

1 tablespoon tahini

To top (your choice): passionfruit, berries, nuts, linseeds (flaxseeds), chia seeds, sunflower seeds and/ or coconut flakes

Whiz all the ingredients except the topping(s) in a high-speed blender until smooth and creamy. Add more milk to thin if necessary.

Share between two bowls and decorate with your chosen topping(s).

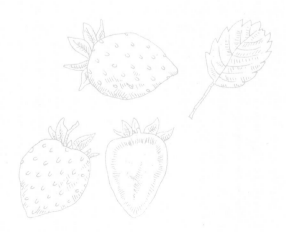

Chocolate and raspberry smoothie bowl

{ *SERVES 2* }

2 frozen bananas

1 ripe avocado, peeled

125 g (4½ oz/1 cup) raspberries

2 tablespoons raw cacao powder

1 teaspoon vanilla powder

130 g (4½ oz/½ cup) sheep's milk yoghurt or Coconut 'Yoghurt' (page 195)

125 ml (4 fl oz/½ cup) almond milk or milk of your choice

To top (your choice): edible flowers, passionfruit, lilly pilly berries, banana, raspberries, blueberries, strawberries, almonds, pepitas (pumpkin seeds), chia seeds, coconut flakes, cacao nibs, granola and/or nut butter

Whiz all the ingredients except the toppings in a high-speed blender until smooth and creamy. The mixture should have a spoonable consistency.

Pour into two bowls and decorate with your chosen topping(s).

MORE SCRUMPTIOUS SMOOTHIE BOWL COMBINATIONS

MACA + CHOCOLATE: frozen banana, coconut milk and maca powder smoothie, topped with nut butter, chia seeds and coconut

PURPLE + CRUNCH: frozen blueberry, spinach, banana and almond milk smoothie, topped with fresh berries and granola

MANGO + OATS: gluten-free oats, coconut milk, banana, sea salt, chia and vanilla smoothie, topped with mango, cacao nibs and mint leaves (make the smoothie the night before for the oats to soak up the liquids and give the smoothie a lovely thick texture)

MATCHA + PEPITAS: matcha tea powder, coconut milk, banana and mint smoothie, topped with pepitas (pumpkin seeds), sliced banana and cacao nibs

PEANUT BUTTER + CHOCOLATE: banana, hazelnut, protein powder, cacao powder and almond milk smoothie, topped with hazelnuts, cacao nibs, pepitas (pumpkin seeds) and coconut flakes

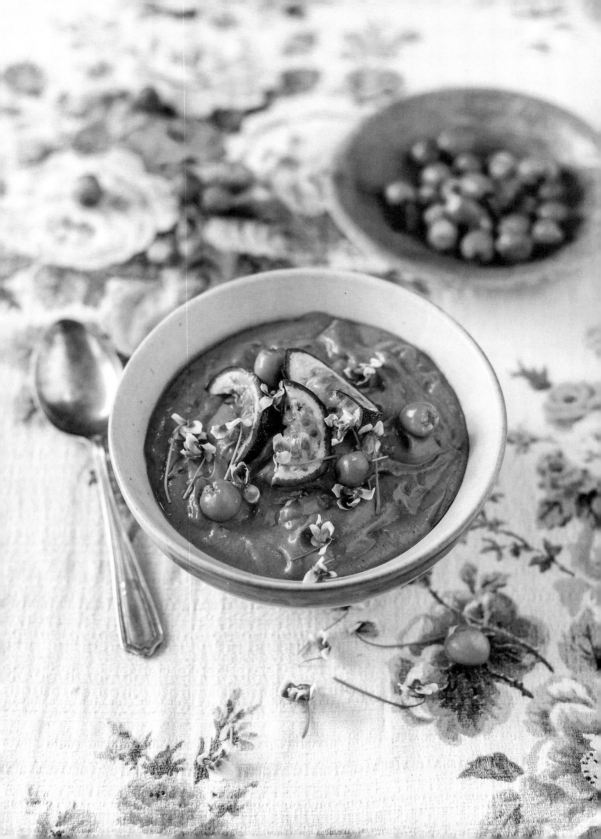

Goji berry and tomato soup

{ *SERVES* 4 }

100 g (3½ oz/1 cup) dried goji berries

filtered water, for soaking

1 tablespoon extra virgin olive oil

1 large brown onion, diced

2 garlic cloves, finely chopped

1 celery stalk, thinly sliced

1 small red chilli, finely chopped

300 g (10½ oz/1½ cups) fresh chopped tomatoes, or 400 g (14 oz) tinned diced tomatoes

1 teaspoon cumin seeds, plus extra to serve

500 ml (17 fl oz/2 cups) vegetable stock

1 tablespoon apple cider vinegar

1 teaspoon grated lemon zest

1 tablespoon lemon juice

handful basil leaves

freshly ground black pepper, to taste

lemon oil (see tip), for drizzling

95 g (3¼ oz/⅓ cup) full-fat plain yoghurt, to serve (optional)

Rinse the goji berries in cold water, then place in a bowl. Cover with filtered water and soak for a few minutes, then drain and set aside. (You can reserve the liquid and use it to replace some of the stock if you like.)

Heat the olive oil in a medium saucepan over medium heat, and sauté the onion, garlic, celery and chilli for 2–3 minutes. Add the tomatoes, goji berries and cumin seeds. Cook for another 3 minutes.

Add the stock, apple cider vinegar, and lemon zest and juice, then bring to the boil. Reduce the heat to low and simmer, covered, for 10 minutes.

Allow to cool slightly, stir in the basil, setting a little aside for a garnish, then purée in a blender until smooth.

Serve garnished with the reserved basil leaves, extra cumin seeds, pepper, a drizzle of lemon oil and a swirl of yoghurt, if using.

SUPERCHARGED TIP

If you don't have lemon oil, mix extra virgin olive oil with a little grated lemon zest.

Lime and mango prawn salad

{ *SERVES* 4 }

Prawns (shrimp) and mango are great pals, and a textbook pairing when it comes to flavour combinations. In Ayurvedic nutrition, mango has properties of sweet and sour, and its quotient of fibre makes it a wonderful laxative for those with a sluggish digestion. Mango can soothe inflamed tissues and has liver-cleansing capabilities due to its diuretic nature.

1 teaspoon ghee

½ teaspoon coriander seeds

½ teaspoon cumin seeds

½ teaspoon garam masala

¼ teaspoon ground turmeric

1 tablespoon lime juice

60 ml (2 fl oz/¼ cup) flaxseed oil

1 tablespoon red onion, finely chopped

pinch of sea salt

1 avocado, peeled and sliced

20 large cooked prawns (shrimp), peeled and deveined

1 large or 2 small mangoes, peeled and grated or finely diced

large handful coriander (cilantro) sprigs

Heat the ghee in a small frying pan over medium heat. Add the spices and swirl to fry for 30 seconds or until fragrant, then transfer to a small bowl to cool.

To the cooled spice mixture, add the lime juice, flaxseed oil and onion, mix with a fork and season with salt.

Arrange the avocado on plates, then top with the prawns and mango. Drizzle the spice mixture over the top, garnish with the coriander and serve.

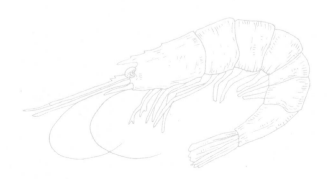

Roasted fig, walnut and goat's cheese salad

{ *SERVES* 4 }

I believe deep down that goat's cheese and beetroot were made for one another. Their romance is proof that opposites attract, and that two entirely different souls can be a match made in heaven. Here, the bright pink, sweet, earthy flavours of beetroot mingle with the rich, creamy tartness of goat's cheese. I highly recommend investing in a quality goat's cheese. It'll be a little extra on your food bill, but it's a decadent treat like no other.

3 small beetroot (beets), peeled and thickly sliced

extra virgin olive oil, for drizzling

6 ripe figs, halved crossways

¼ teaspoon ground cinnamon

apple cider vinegar, for drizzling

100 g (3½ oz) walnuts

200 g (7 oz) English spinach, plus extra to serve (optional)

100 g (3½ oz) goat's cheese

juice of ½ lemon

2 thyme sprigs

freshly ground black pepper

microherbs, to serve (optional)

1 orange, sliced and roasted, to serve (optional)

Preheat the oven to 220°C (425°F).

Toss the beetroot in a roasting tray with a drizzle of olive oil. Roast for 25 minutes, or until just softened. Remove the tray, lay the fig halves, cut side up, around the beetroot then sprinkle with the cinnamon and drizzle over some olive oil and apple cider vinegar. Roast for 5 minutes then add the walnuts and cook for a further 5 minutes, or until the figs are golden, plump and slightly softened. Allow to cool to room temperature.

Put the spinach on a platter or in a salad bowl, add the figs and walnuts, and crumble over the goat's cheese. Drizzle with olive oil and the lemon juice. Top with the thyme, a grind or two of black pepper, some microherbs, extra spinach and roasted orange slices, if using.

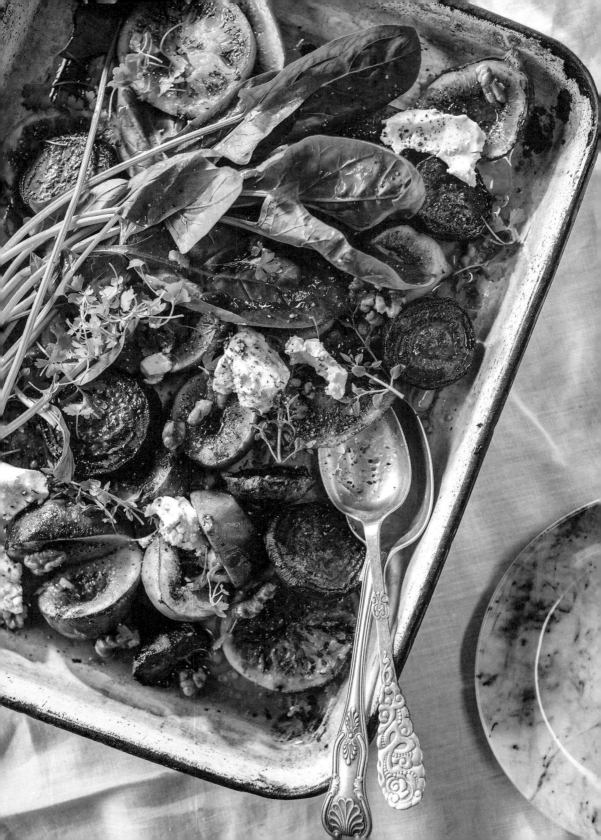

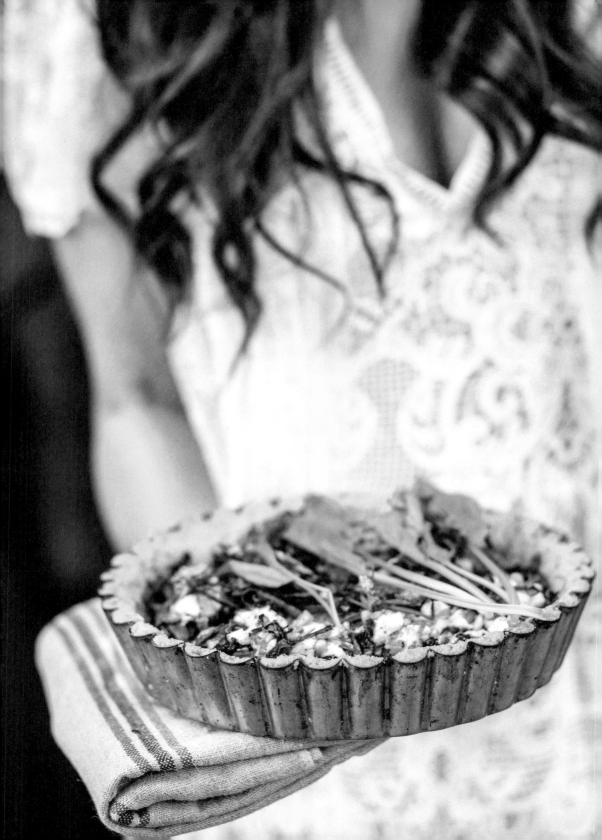

Spinach, goat's cheese and pine nut tart

{ *SERVES* 4 }

This tart is a trusty friend when you want to take something simple but special along to a potluck feast or lunchtime communal gathering. Its gluten-free almond crust, filled with the flavours of creamy goat's cheese, cumin, nutmeg and earthy pine nuts, just beckons to be shared with others. A beautiful recipe to extend love through food.

Crust

300 g (10½ oz/3 cups) almond meal

1 teaspoon bicarbonate of soda (baking soda)

1 teaspoon dried rosemary

125 ml (4 fl oz/½ cup) extra virgin olive oil or melted butter

2 tablespoons cold filtered water

Filling

2 tablespoons olive oil

3 brown onions, very thinly sliced

3 garlic cloves, crushed

500 g (1 lb 2 oz) English spinach, washed and chopped (can use frozen)

¼ teaspoon freshly grated nutmeg

1 teaspoon ground cumin

sea salt and freshly ground black pepper, to taste

4 eggs, whisked

200 g (7 oz) goat's cheese, crumbled into large chunks

2 tablespoons raw honey (optional)

50 g (1¾ oz/⅓ cup) pine nuts

Preheat the oven to 180°C (350°F) and lightly grease a 22 cm (8½ inch) loose-based flan (tart) tin.

To make the crust, combine the almond meal, bicarbonate of soda and rosemary in a large bowl and mix well. In a separate bowl, whisk the olive oil with half the water. Stir the olive oil and water into the dry ingredients and mix well to combine. If the mixture is too dry, add more of the water. Spoon the mixture into the prepared tin and spread evenly over the base and up the sides. Bake for 10 minutes.

Meanwhile, to prepare the filling, heat the oil in a large saucepan and fry the onions for 6–7 minutes, until browned and caramelised. Add the garlic and cook for 1 minute, then remove from the heat and set aside.

Place the spinach in a large bowl and pour over boiling water. Allow to cool, then use your hands to wring it out until as dry as possible.

In a large bowl, mix the spinach, onions and garlic, nutmeg and cumin, then season with salt and pepper. Mix in the egg, half the goat's cheese and the honey, if using. Spoon the mixture into the crust, crumble over the remaining goat's cheese and scatter over the pine nuts. Bake for 15–20 minutes, until the crust, cheese and nuts are golden.

Kakadu plum and blueberry ice cream

{ *SERVES* 2 }

Kakadu plum, also known as gubinge, is a native fruit from the Kimberley region in Western Australia that has been enjoyed by Indigenous Australians for thousands of years. It's one of the highest real-food sources of vitamin C known, and has an astringent, citrusy flavour.

2 frozen bananas

155 g (5½ oz/1 cup) frozen blueberries

60 ml (2 fl oz/¼ cup) chilled coconut milk, plus extra as needed

1 teaspoon kakadu plum (gubinge) powder

1 teaspoon alcohol-free vanilla extract

mint leaves and pistachio nut kernels, to serve

Whiz all the ingredients except the mint and pistachios in a food processor until creamy, adding more coconut milk if needed for a smooth consistency.

Serve in two bowls, garnished with mint leaves and pistachio nuts. For the best taste, eat immediately.

Mango, lime and saffron tapioca pudding

{ *SERVES* 2–3 }

1.25 litres (44 fl oz/5 cups) filtered water

75 g (2¾ oz/½ cup) pearl tapioca

170 ml (5½ fl oz/⅔ cup) coconut milk

⅛ teaspoon saffron threads, crushed

¼ teaspoon sea salt

¾ teaspoon grated lime zest

1 teaspoon lime juice

½ teaspoon alcohol-free vanilla extract or powder

6 drops liquid stevia

15 g (½ oz/¼ cup) coconut flakes

1 ripe mango, peeled and diced

Bring the water to the boil in a medium saucepan over medium heat, then stir in the tapioca, reduce the heat to low and cook for 15 minutes, or until the tapioca is translucent and cooked through.

In a large bowl, whisk the coconut milk with the saffron, salt, lime zest and juice, vanilla and stevia. Add this mixture along with the coconut flakes to the tapioca, and continue cooking over low heat for a further 10 minutes, stirring frequently.

Spoon into bowls and top with the mango.

Fruit sorbets four ways

{ *SERVES* 2 }

Mango and lime

185 g (6½ oz) frozen mango pieces

60 ml (2 fl oz/¼ cup) coconut water

zest of ½ lime

1 tablespoon lime juice

Banana and coconut

130 g (4½ oz/1 cup) frozen banana slices

60 ml (2 fl oz/¼ cup) coconut milk

Berry and lemon

220 g (7¾ oz/1 cup) frozen mixed berries

60 ml (2 fl oz/¼ cup) coconut water

grated zest of ½ lemon

1 tablespoon lemon juice

Mint choc chip

1 frozen peeled and sliced avocado

60 ml (2 fl oz/¼ cup) coconut water

½ teaspoon peppermint extract

½ teaspoon cacao nibs, plus extra to serve

For each sorbet, whiz all the ingredients in a blender until smooth (see tip), then serve immediately or freeze for 3–4 hours to harden.

SUPERCHARGED TIP

If you don't have a high-speed blender, add extra liquid to get it moving along.

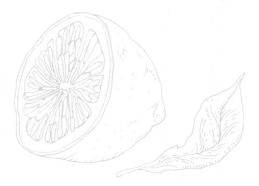

Sea salt, fresh raspberry and slivered almond chocolate

{ *MAKES ABOUT 150 G [5½ OZ]* }

Life's too short not to savour the divine sensation that chocolate brings. And this sea salt, slivered almond and fresh raspberry delight is a super-romantic treat, perfect for Valentine's Day or when trying to impress a special someone. The addition of sea salt to home-made chocolate is a must, and seems to lift the point of sweet bliss to new heights.

60 g (2¼ oz) coconut butter

2 tablespoons coconut oil

55 g (2 oz/¼ cup) grated cacao butter

1 heaped tablespoon raw cacao powder

2 tablespoons rice malt syrup or 1 teaspoon stevia powder

generous pinch of sea salt

1 teaspoon alcohol-free vanilla extract

2 tablespoons natural peanut butter (optional)

handful raspberries, halved

handful slivered almonds, toasted

Line a baking tray with baking paper.

Melt the coconut butter, coconut oil and cacao butter in a bowl sitting over (but not touching) a bowl of very hot water and whisk to combine. Add the cacao powder, rice malt syrup, salt, vanilla and peanut butter, if using, and whisk to combine.

Pour into the prepared tray and scatter over the raspberries and almonds. Place in the freezer for at least 30 minutes, or until solid. Remove from the freezer and break into shards or chop into squares. Store in an airtight container in the freezer.

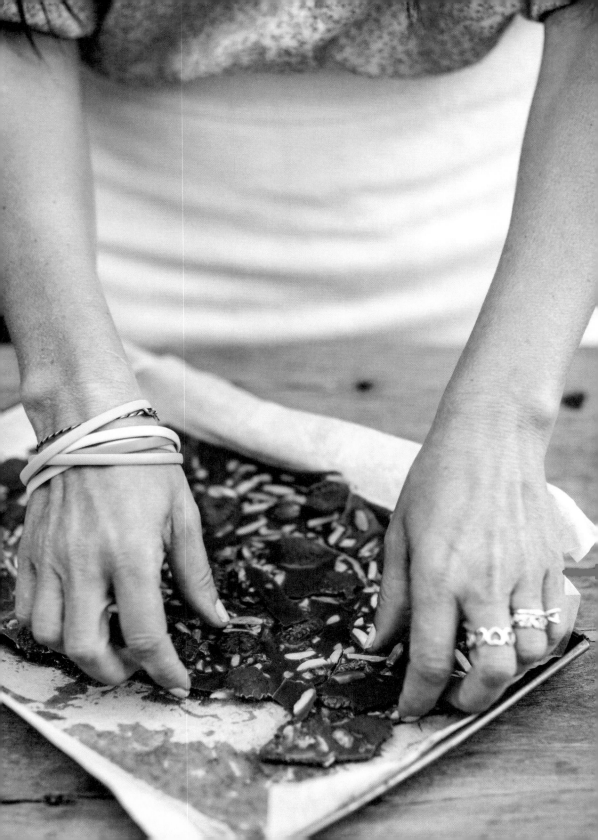

Building your spice rack

One of the first places to begin your kitchen adventure and love affair with food and ingredients is your humble spice rack. It can rapidly become your most loyal supporter in the kitchen.

A spice rack serves as a kaleidoscopic palette of flavoursome dried herbs and spices that will impart specific flavours to your cooking. These spices can be paired or used on their own to complement your culinary creations.

To set up a do-it-yourself spice rack or spice drawer, it all comes down to the space you have in your kitchen and what will be most practical for you. Many homeware stores sell rectangular storage baskets that can slide in and out of your pantry or cupboards and be filled with spices.

You could also recycle a wooden box as a home for your spice collection. You could keep the spices in their original packaging, and if they're in packets invest in some kitchen storage bag clips to reseal them after opening. This will stop any spills that make your cupboards smell like a curry house!

If you have plenty of shelf space or a large walk-in pantry, you could dedicate a shelf to spices, using small screw-top preserving jars or little spring-clip jars for storage. This is an ideal way to store spices, as it saves you fiddling through a spice box or drawer, which can become disorganised very easily. Because my kitchen is the hub of my home and I spend a lot of time creating recipes, I have all my spices in alphabetical order for ease of use, but you don't have to go that far!

A handy thing to do is buy a jar for every spice you use, and use a labeller or a permanent marker to clearly indicate which spice is which. Many spices are a similar colour, so good labelling will save you a lot of time trying to find what you need.

Having your spices in glass jars will allow you to see which ones you need to top up before they actually run out. Depending on the way you like your kitchen to look, stacked rows of jars along a shelf can be both stylish and practical.

MY GO-TO SPICES

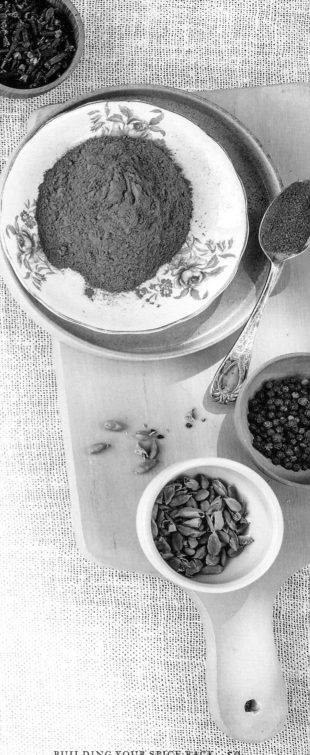

{ Cloves }

QUALITY: Spicy and pungent.

USE: Ground and whole to add complexity to apple crumbles and brown rice puddings, or combined with other spices to complement curries.

{ Cinnamon }

QUALITY: Spicy and sweet.

USE: Ground and whole sticks in sweet or savoury dishes. Excellent blood-sugar stabiliser.

{ Paprika }

QUALITY: Hot and sweet.

USE: Depending on the heat when ground, will add sweetness and varying levels of heat to savoury dishes.

{ Black peppercorns }

QUALITY: Hot and pungent.

USE: Whole in soups, stocks or chai; ground over meals with sea salt.

{ Cardamom }

QUALITY: Citrusy, spicy and sweet.

USE: Whole pods are wonderful bruised and added to curries, soups, dhal, chai and sweet foods.

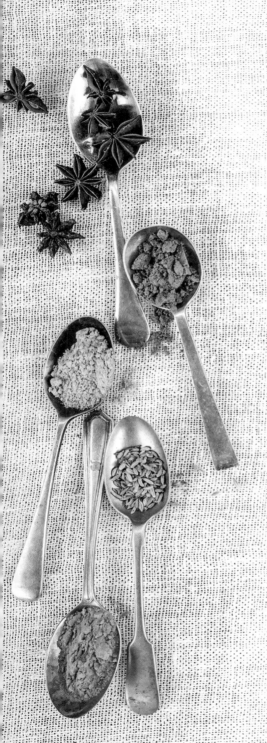

{ Star anise }

QUALITY: Licorice.

USE: Beautiful in Asian creations, particularly those with pork or chicken. A primary ingredient in Chinese five-spice.

{ Cumin }

QUALITY: Earthy and musky.

USE: Offers flavour and aroma to a variety of meals. Can be used ground, or as whole seeds for a more pronounced pop of flavour.

{ Ginger }

QUALITY: Citrusy and warming.

USE: Lovely in chai, used on its own to make an anti-inflammatory tea, or as a warming spice added to sweet and savoury dishes. Imparts the most flavour when used fresh, but can also be used ground.

{ Fennel seeds }

QUALITY: Licorice or aniseed.

USE: To flavour breads, curries, meat and vegetable dishes, or in yoghurt-based dips such as raita. You'll get the most flavour out of these darlings by dry-frying then pounding using a mortar and pestle.

{ Turmeric }

QUALITY: Earthy and pungent.

USE: A potent anti-inflammatory that can be used to make healing teas, or added to curries, meat and noodle dishes. Pairs wonderfully with coconut.

{ Bay leaf }

QUALITY: Herbal and floral.

USE: Brings out the best in warm spices and meaty flavours in soups, stews and stocks.

{ Saffron }

QUALITY: Grassy, honey tones.

USE: A tiny amount of these expensive golden threads can be used anywhere vanilla would be; classically used in Middle Eastern dishes. Pairs well with light meats and vegetables such as cauliflower.

{ Nutmeg }

QUALITY: Spicy and piquant.

USE: Freshly grated or ground, pairs well with sweet potatoes and creamy vegetable bakes, or with meats such as lamb or pork. Lovely with creamy soups or cheesy flavours. Adds depth and an earthy balance to creamy desserts such as rice pudding and custards.

{ Coriander seed }

QUALITY: Floral and nutty.

USE: Gorgeous in curries, soups or stews. Contains essential volatile oils responsible for its digestive and carminative (gas-relieving) properties.

{ Cayenne pepper }

QUALITY: Hot and spicy.

USE: Adds a layer of clean, hot spice to savoury meals. Aids in thermo-genesis (energy use to digest food) making it a great fat-burning food.

{ Vanilla bean }

QUALITY: Sweet, floral and fruity.

USE: In sweet baked goods, pancakes, porridges and desserts.

HERBS AND SPICES

Mixing and mingling herbs and adding a sprig or two to your diet can enhance your meals no end, both culinarily and medicinally. Herbs really are a dream come true in the kitchen, and I use their aromas to enliven the simplest of recipes. To find out more about growing your own herb garden, head over to page 211.

Harmonising with fresh herbs will offer you an insight into their prowess: readily releasing their beautiful perfumed flavours into your dishes. You'll frequently find me hobnobbing with highly fragrant herbs. I fraternise with fennel for its fragrant flavourings and anti-inflammatory and digestive capabilities. Antibacterial basil is also a wonderful anti-inflammatory herb.

It's easy to buy a bunch of fresh herbs, use only a couple of leaves in a recipe, then shove them to the back of the fridge and forget about them, only to find them later all limp and bedraggled. When storing herbs, the hardy ones like rosemary, thyme and sage can stay aromatic for up to two weeks in the fridge, but do remember to keep them as dry as possible. The best place to do this is usually the top shelf.

Generally speaking, the golden rule when cooking with herbs is fat first, herbs last. I've infused many of the recipes in this book with delicious herbs and spices, and I'd like to draw your attention to some of my favourites.

If the thought of herbs and spices gets you into a muddle, and tarragon and oregano sound like American states, I've also created a wonderful online reference guide, including all of the most common and some uncommon herbs and spices, at superchargedfood.com.

You'll soon find that using herbs can be the difference between you and your family pushing your plates away and eating your meals with delight.

{ Asafoetida }

Native to the deserts of Iran and mountains of Afghanistan, asafoetida is a standard component of South Indian and Maharashtrian cuisine. Known for its strong leek-like odour, this pungent spice will make a tasty addition to your next curry or lentil dish. The medicinal spice is used as a digestive aid, to prevent overgrowth of gas-producing bacteria in the gut microflora, thus helping to reduce flatulence. It is also used as an antiviral to fight off flu.

{ Basil }

Highly aromatic, with a robust licorice flavour, basil is commonly used fresh in recipes, as cooking can quickly destroy its flavour. It's superb in a pesto or as a finishing touch on pasta dishes. My favourite is scattering fresh basil leaves over a caprese salad for a refreshing Italian dish. Rehydrate with my Lemon, Strawberry and Basil Water Jar (page 247).

{ Cardamom }

Made from the seeds of several plants native to India, Nepal, Pakistan and Bhutan, cardamom provides a warm, aromatic flavour that's widely used in Indian cuisine. Found in black or green seed varieties, cardamom is commonly used in baked goods, delivering a delightful flavour when used in combination with spices such as clove and cinnamon.

{ Cinnamon }

A versatile spice found in almost every world cuisine and used in both sweet and savoury dishes, cinnamon is also a great spice for jazzing up your morning porridge, sprinkling over your fruit salad or even livening up your tea. Known for helping to balance blood sugar and cholesterol levels, cinnamon has also been found to stimulate digestion and appetite, soothe an upset stomach, relieve indigestion and improve circulation. Delivering a large dose of antioxidants, cinnamon is a regular star on my kitchen shelf. Create a stack of blueberry pancakes with a chai coconut cream. Or whip up my tummy-warming Macacino (page 172).

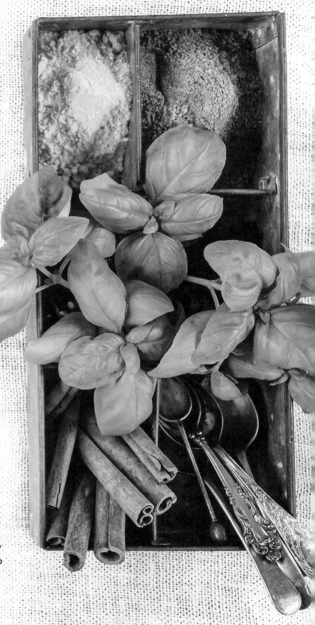

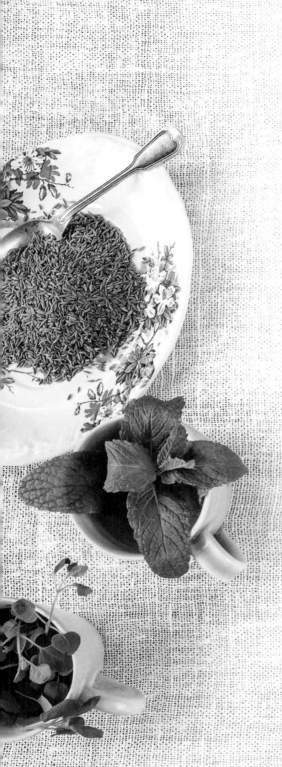

{ Cumin }

Native to the eastern Mediterranean and India, cumin is a smoky and earthy spice used in Mexican, North African, Middle Eastern and Indian cuisines. This medicinal spice is known to aid digestive problems, including diarrhoea, colic and gas. Use it in a creamy dressing over a daikon (mooli) and endive salad.

{ Fennel seed }

With its sweet, licorice-like flavour, fennel seed has long been revered as a sacred herb for its health benefits. Popular in Mediterranean, Indian and Middle Eastern cuisines, it makes a tasty addition to meat dishes and casseroles, and can be chewed on its own as a breath freshener or digestion aid. It is also wonderful in home-made baked beans.

{ Mint }

The leaves of this surprisingly versatile, intensely flavoured herb have a warm, fresh, aromatic, sweet flavour with a cool aftertaste, and are used in both sweet and savoury dishes. Try mint paired with lamb, peas and potatoes. Or use it in a mint sauce, in teas and beverages, or with ice cream or chocolate. There are so many ways you can have fun with this sweet little herb! Be charmed and calmed by the mango and oats variation of my Smoothie Bowl (page 46).

{ Oregano }

This important culinary herb can often be more flavourful when dried. It has a robust, warm and slightly bitter taste. Called the 'pizza herb' when World War II soldiers took the flavour back with them to the United States, its most prominent use is as a staple in Italian cuisine. Oregano is delicious with roasted or grilled vegetables, meats and fish, and charming in a salad or sprinkled over ripe sliced tomatoes with sea salt and a drizzle of extra virgin olive oil. It will have your family's tastebuds standing to attention. I use it in my Supercharged Shakshuka (page 68).

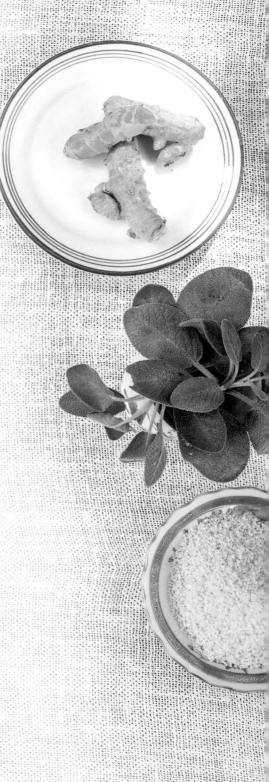

{ Turmeric }

The ground or grated rootstalk of a tropical
plant in the ginger family, turmeric is one
of my favourites thanks to its powerful
anti-inflammatory properties. Sometimes used
more for its colour than its pungent flavour, this
bright golden spice has a mild and woody aroma.
It's perfect for pilafs and other rice dishes,
curries, soups and lentil dishes; I adore adding
it to my curries and chicken casseroles.

{ Sage }

For generations, sage has been used in
Britain as an essential herb, along with
parsley, rosemary and thyme. Sage is often
found in northern Italian cooking, such as the
classic saltimbocca, and its pine-like flavour
is delicious in breads and vegetable bakes,
and used to flavour meats. Sage is known
to enhance memory and may provide some
benefit to Alzheimer's sufferers. It also reduces
inflammation and is a potent antioxidant. It
can even help lower cholesterol and has been
traditionally used by menopausal women to
ease hot flushes. Quite an all-rounder! If you've
never tried sage, you may find the aroma quite
distinctive, so start with small portions and add
to your liking. My Mushroom and Kale Lasagne
(page 304) is a quick and easy dish to add to
the family's weekly meal plan.

{ Salt }

Always stock some good-quality sea salt (such as
Celtic) or pink Himalayan salt, which you'll find
are packed full of minerals to add even more
nutrition and great flavour to your cooking.

Peanut butter and turmeric smoothie

{ *SERVES* 1 }

Peanut butter brings back nostalgic feelings of mischief and giggles during recess in primary school, while we hungrily devoured our staple peanut butter sandwiches. I always favoured the crunchy variety and still enjoy the flavours as an adult. This quirky smoothie combines my childhood favourite with creamy sweet bananas, an exotic twist of golden turmeric, and sex-drive-boosting maca powder for the grown-ups.

250 ml (9 fl oz/1 cup) almond or coconut milk, or your milk of choice

1 frozen banana

1 heaped tablespoon natural peanut butter or other nut butter

1 teaspoon maca powder (optional)

½ teaspoon ground turmeric

pinch of sea salt

pinch of ground cinnamon, to serve

Whiz all the ingredients except the cinnamon in a high-speed blender or food processor until smooth. Pour into a glass, sprinkle the cinnamon on top and serve.

Curried mixed nuts

{ *MAKES* 420 G [14¾ OZ / 3 CUPS] }

420 g (14¾ oz/3 cups) mixed nuts (e.g. blanched almonds, macadamia nuts, cashews, pecans)

2 tablespoons rice malt syrup

2 teaspoons curry powder

1 teaspoon ground cinnamon

¼ teaspoon ground cumin

1 teaspoon sea salt

Preheat the oven to 180°C (350°F) and line a baking tray with baking paper.

Put all the ingredients in a large bowl and mix with a spoon until the nuts are well coated.

Spread the nuts over the prepared baking tray and bake for 12–15 minutes, stirring frequently to ensure they don't burn. They should be crisp and lightly coloured.

Allow to cool before serving.

Spicy kale with toasted seeds

{ *SERVES* 3 }

If you're after a stand-out vegetable option that provides a mountain of fibre, iron, and vitamins A, C and K, look no further. Bursting with character and flavour, kale has a wonderful nutritional profile that combines antioxidants with anti-inflammatory and detoxifying properties. If you're going to consume large quantities of kale, it's best to eat it cooked.

1 tablespoon ghee

4 handfuls kale leaves, spines removed, washed, dried and roughly chopped

½ teaspoon black mustard seeds

½ teaspoon ground coriander

¼ teaspoon asafoetida powder

4 small green chillies, finely chopped

1 × 2 cm (¾ in) piece fresh ginger, finely chopped

1 garlic clove, chopped

coriander (cilantro) leaves, to serve

40 g (1½ oz/⅓ cup) toasted seeds (e.g. sesame, sunflower)

Heat half the ghee in a large frying pan or wok over medium heat, add the kale to wilt in batches, then set aside.

Heat the remaining ghee in the same pan over medium heat, add the mustard seeds and sizzle for 1 minute. Add the ground coriander, asafoetida powder, chilli and ginger. Fry for 1 minute, then add the garlic and kale. Cook, stirring, for 2–3 minutes.

Pile into a serving dish and scatter over some coriander leaves and the toasted seeds.

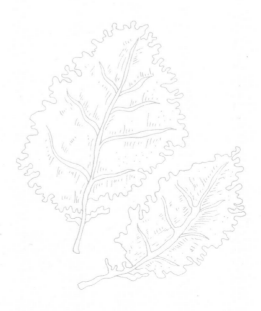

Supercharged shakshuka

{ *SERVES* 4 }

2 tablespoons extra virgin olive
  oil, plus extra for drizzling

1 brown onion, halved and
  thinly sliced

1 large capsicum (pepper),
  seeded and thinly sliced

3 garlic cloves, thinly sliced

1 teaspoon ground cumin

1 teaspoon sweet paprika, plus
  extra to serve

pinch of cayenne pepper,
  or to taste

1 teaspoon dried oregano

400 g (14 oz/2 cups) chopped
  tomatoes or 400 g (14 oz)
  tinned diced tomatoes

1 tablespoon wheat-free tamari
  or coconut aminos

45 g (1½ oz/1 cup) baby English
  spinach leaves, plus extra
  to serve

pinch of sea salt

freshly ground black pepper,
  to taste

4 large eggs

150 g (5½ oz/1¼ cups)
  crumbled goat's cheese

snipped chives, to serve

edible flowers, to serve
  (optional)

Preheat the oven to 190°C (375°F).

Heat the olive oil in a large heavy-based ovenproof frying pan over medium–low heat and sauté the onion and capsicum for 3–4 minutes, until soft. Add the garlic, spices and oregano, then cook for 1 minute. Add the tomatoes, tamari and spinach, season with salt and pepper, then cook for 4–5 minutes, until the sauce has thickened.

Make four indentations in the mixture with a spoon and carefully crack in the eggs. Transfer to the oven and bake for 10–15 minutes, until the eggs are set.

Scatter over the goat's cheese, chives, extra spinach and flowers, if using, sprinkle over extra paprika and pepper, and drizzle with extra olive oil. Serve immediately.

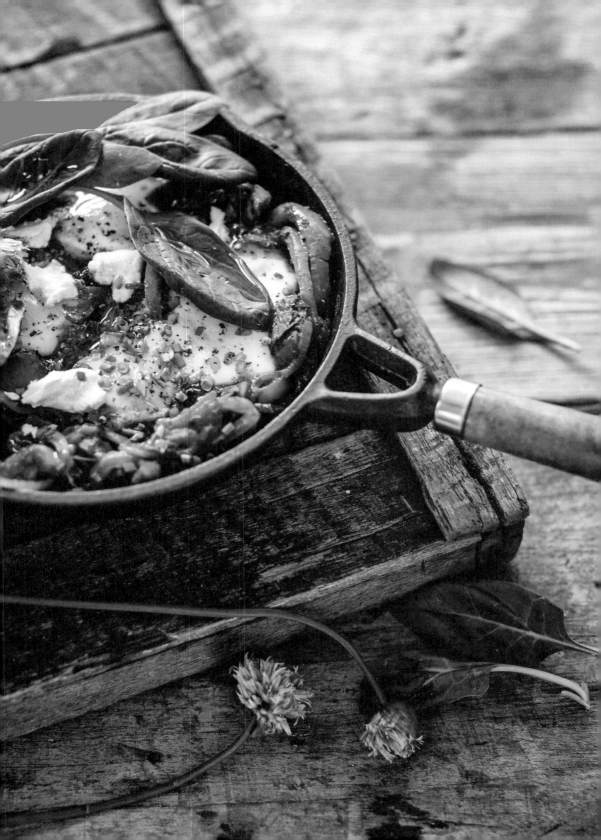

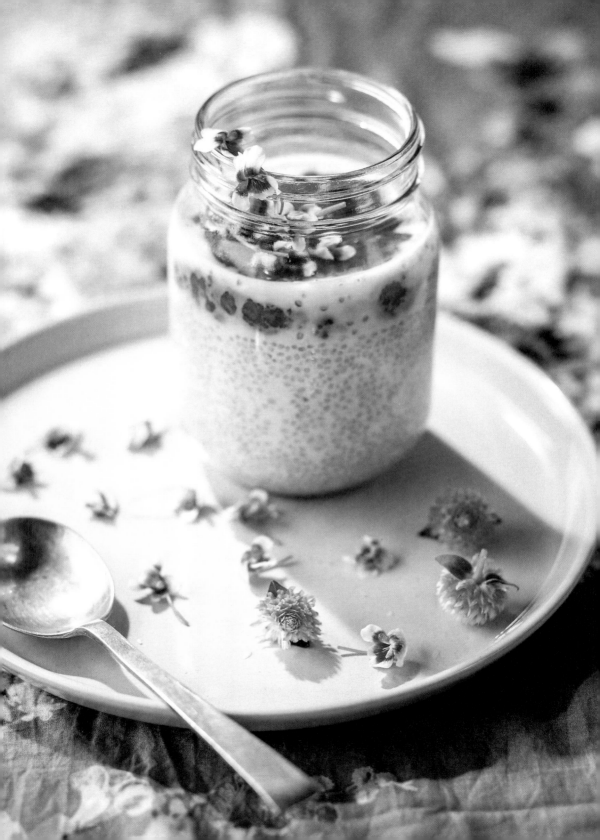

Sweet berry spiced chia pudding

{ SERVES 2 }

45 g (1½ oz/⅓ cup) white chia
seeds

500 ml (17 fl oz/2 cups) coconut
milk

1 teaspoon alcohol-free vanilla
extract

10 drops liquid stevia or your
sweetener of choice

220 g (7¾ oz/1 cup) mixed
berries

1 cinnamon stick

1 star anise

filtered water, as needed

edible flowers, ground
cinnamon or star anise,
to serve (optional)

Mix the chia seeds with the coconut milk,
vanilla and stevia, then divide between two
screw-top jars or bowls. Seal tightly and
refrigerate for 6 hours or overnight.

Put the berries in a small saucepan with the
cinnamon stick, star anise and a little filtered
water. Bring to the boil over medium heat,
then reduce the heat to low and simmer
for 2–3 minutes, until reduced to a jam-like
consistency, adding a little more water if
necessary. Allow to cool slightly, then add
to the top of the puddings.

Top with edible flowers, ground cinnamon or
star anise, if using.

SUPERCHARGED TIP
The puddings will keep in the fridge for up to
3 days.

Turmeric seeded loaf

{ MAKES 9 x 30 CM [3½ x 12 INCH] LOAF }

200 g (7 oz/2 cups) almond
meal

60 g (2¼ oz/½ cup) walnuts

50 g (1¾ oz/½ cup) flaked
almonds

75 g (2¾ oz/½ cup) pepitas
(pumpkin seeds)

40 g (1½ oz/¼ cup) sunflower
seeds

¼ teaspoon salt

1 teaspoon ground turmeric

½ teaspoon gluten-free baking
powder

15 g (½ oz/¼ cup) coconut
flakes

3 eggs

2 egg whites

90 g (3¼ oz) butter or coconut
oil, melted

2 tablespoons rice malt syrup

½ banana, mashed

Preheat the oven to 170°C (325°F) and line
a 9 × 30 cm (3½ × 12 inch) loaf (bar) tin with
baking paper.

Combine the almond meal, nuts, seeds, salt,
turmeric, baking powder and coconut flakes
in a large bowl.

In a small bowl, whisk together the remaining
ingredients. Add the wet mixture to the dry
and mix until well combined.

Pour the batter into the prepared tin and bake
for 45–50 minutes, until a skewer inserted in
the centre comes out clean.

Allow to cool in the tin before slicing.

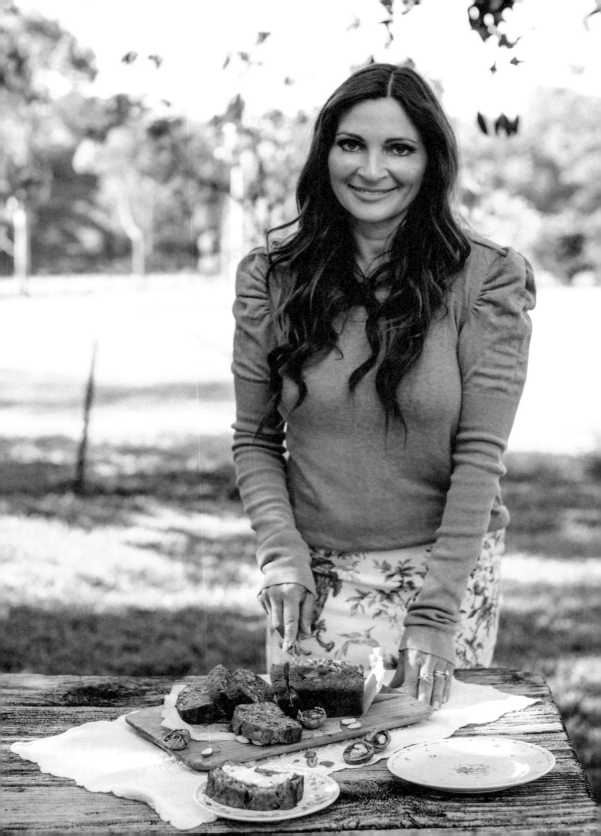

Meatball stew

{ SERVES 3–4 }

The best way to enjoy this comforting meatball stew is by using the freshest ingredients possible, including a home-made stock or broth for a purer and deeper flavour.

1 red capsicum (pepper), seeded and finely chopped

1 small red onion, finely chopped

3 garlic cloves, finely chopped

6 olives, pitted and chopped

1 red chilli, seeded and finely chopped (optional)

500 g (1 lb 2 oz) minced (ground) beef or lamb

2 eggs

50 g (1³/₄ oz/¹/₂ cup) almond meal or ground cashews

2 teaspoons ground cumin

1 tablespoon paprika

sea salt and freshly ground black pepper, to taste

2 tablespoons coconut oil

2 carrots, finely chopped

2 celery stalks, thinly sliced

1 turnip, diced

500 ml (17 fl oz/2 cups) beef or chicken stock (see tip)

400 g (14 oz/2 cups) chopped tomatoes or 400 g (14 oz) tinned diced tomatoes

2 tablespoons coconut aminos

1 teaspoon grated lime zest

1 tablespoon lime juice

coriander (cilantro) leaves, to serve

1 avocado, peeled and sliced

coconut milk, to serve (optional)

Combine the capsicum, onion, garlic, olives and chilli in a bowl, then stir in the meat, eggs, almond meal, spices, and some salt and pepper. Using your hands, roll the mixture into walnut-sized balls.

Heat half the coconut oil in a large saucepan over medium heat and sauté the carrot, celery and turnip for about 10 minutes, until golden. Add the stock, tomatoes, coconut aminos and lime zest and juice, bring to the boil, then reduce the heat to low and simmer for 10–15 minutes, until the vegetables are cooked.

Meanwhile, heat the remaining oil in a frying pan over medium–high heat and, working in batches if necessary, brown the meatballs all over. Reduce the heat to low, cover, and simmer the meatballs in their own juices for 15–20 minutes, until cooked through.

Share the meatballs between bowls, ladle over the vegetable stew and garnish with coriander, avocado slices and a dash of coconut milk, if using.

SUPERCHARGED TIP

If you don't have time to cook up the broth yourself, many butchers now offer broths, and high-quality additive-free packaged versions are also available.

Turmeric cauliflower rice

{ *SERVES* 2-4 }

1 head cauliflower

2 tablespoons olive oil, or coconut oil, melted

2 teaspoons ground turmeric

10 g (^{1}/$_4$ oz/^{1}/$_4$ cup) nutritional yeast flakes

To serve (optional)

large handful basil leaves, chopped

handful mint leaves, torn

75 g (2^3/$_4$ oz/^{1}/$_2$ cup) dried cranberries

1 teaspoon grated lemon zest

60 ml (2 fl oz/^{1}/$_4$ cup) lemon juice

sea salt and freshly ground black pepper, to taste

olive oil, for drizzling

Preheat the oven to 220°C (425°F) and line a baking tray with baking paper.

Break the cauliflower into florets, discarding the stems. Working in batches, pulse the florets in a food processor until they resemble rice. Transfer to a large bowl, and add the olive oil, turmeric and yeast flakes. Mix, ensuring the 'rice' is well coated.

Spread in a single layer on the prepared baking tray and bake, stirring once or twice, for about 25 minutes, until starting to crisp and colour.

Use immediately as a side dish or dress it up by stirring in basil, mint, cranberries, lemon zest and juice, and seasoning with salt and pepper. Drizzle over olive oil to serve.

Cinnamon and rhubarb cake

{ *SERVES 6-8* }

60 g (2¼ oz) unsalted butter, softened

1 teaspoon grated lemon zest

225 g (8 oz/1½ cups) coconut sugar

2 eggs

200 g (7 oz/2 cups) almond meal

½ teaspoon gluten-free baking powder

1 teaspoon bicarbonate of soda (baking soda)

1 teaspoon ground cinnamon

½ teaspoon freshly grated nutmeg

¼ teaspoon sea salt

125 ml (4 fl oz/½ cup) coconut cream

250 g (9 oz/2 cups) chopped rhubarb (see tip)

Preheat the oven to 170°C (325°F). Grease an 18 cm (7 inch) round cake tin or a 9 × 30 cm (3½ × 12 inch) loaf (bar) tin.

In a large bowl, beat the butter, lemon zest, coconut sugar and eggs until creamy. Fold in the almond meal, baking powder, bicarbonate of soda, cinnamon, nutmeg, salt and coconut cream. Gently fold in the rhubarb.

Spoon the mixture into the prepared tin and bake for 45–55 minutes, until the cake springs back when pressed in the centre. Cool in the tin for 10 minutes, then turn out onto a wire rack to cool completely.

SUPERCHARGED TIP

If using a loaf tin, you can lay the rhubarb, unchopped, on top of the cake rather than stirring it through chopped. Brush the rhubarb and the top of the cake with warmed honey or rice malt syrup for a lovely glazed finish.

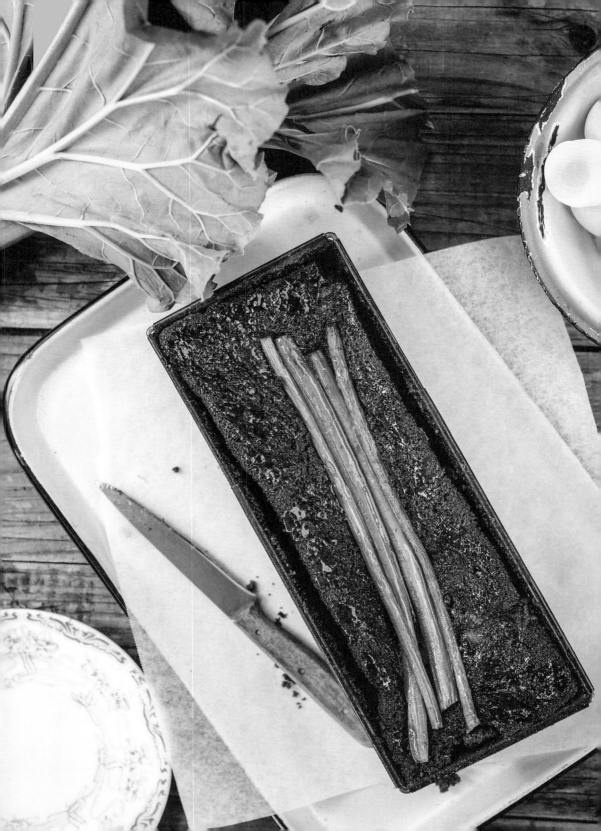

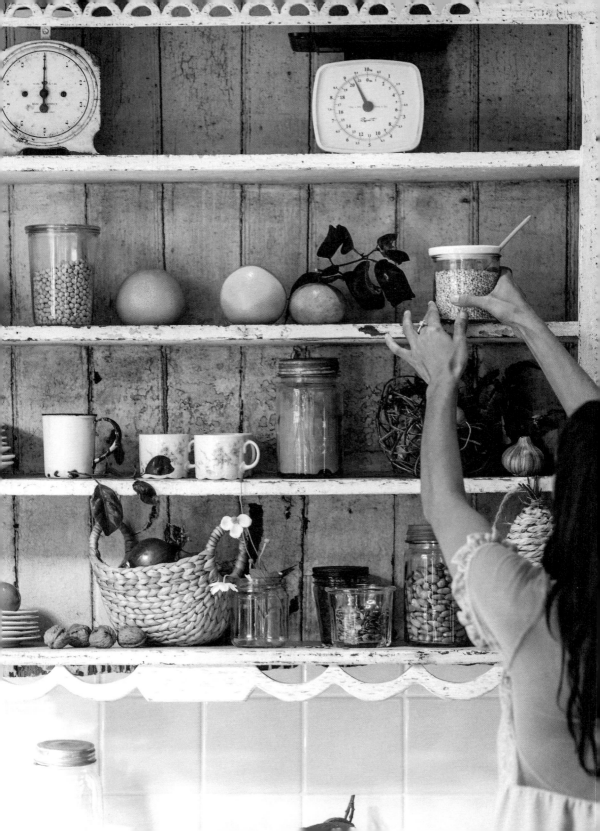

Stocking your pantry, fridge and freezer

When transforming your kitchen into a supercharged paradise equipped for serving up fulfilling and tantalising meals, work on getting a few basics in place. Stock your pantry with essentials that bring oodles of flavour and texture to your dishes. Not only will this turn them into enticing meals your whole family will enjoy, but knowing everything is ready to go will also make it simpler and faster to get cracking, saving you time and energy.

A well-stocked pantry, fridge and freezer are critical tools for planning ahead. Getting your pantry right and always having the basics on hand means fewer trips to the supermarket in the long run, and smaller trips where you'll just be topping up your perishable items – which is better for your purse strings and the environment.

PANTRY

Along with your spice rack (see page 58), build up your pantry slowly and systematically, and focus on dry goods and staples. Try keeping the following fundamentals in your pantry.

Flavour providers

Onions and garlic, both from the *Allium* genus of plants, are two of my favourite flavour accompaniments to use in cooking. They don't just play an important culinary role, they also provide a plethora of health benefits.

When you start by sautéing onion or garlic at the beginning of cooking, you'll find they unleash a powerful flavour that helps release the aromas of the other ingredients in your dish. This is a really important first step, as the strong flavour combinations will only increase the longer you wait to eat it. This is perfect for dishes you plan to reheat the following day.

Onions can stay fresh for well over a month in your pantry, and garlic can last for more than three months, so you'll have your flavour friends right by your side for a good length of time.

Grains and seeds

An absolute staple, grains and seeds are among the most affordable ingredients you can add to any meal. Use brown rice, quinoa and buckwheat to create hearty and nourishing dishes. Each one is versatile, budget-friendly and will last for months sealed in a jar in your pantry.

If you plan to reheat a dish, add some brown rice to bulk it up and allow it to serve a larger group of people – and at the same time make it even more affordable. Repurposing last night's roast meat or vegetables into a fried rice is super-fast and makes for a tasty and convenient work lunch. Brown rice is full of fibre and a great way to satisfy your tummy.

Teff and quinoa have become more popular over the last few years and are two of the more affordable and versatile 'powerfoods' of today. There are a bunch of delicious teff and quinoa recipes in this book, and their versatility can transport you from breakfast to dinner.

Buckwheat has also become a go-to grain substitute in recent times, and is a scrumptious alternative to rice or can be made into porridge for a warming winter breakfast. If you're feeling adventurous, try scattering some buckwheat grains over your berries or yoghurt for added texture.

Oaten porridge is a perfect way to start a cold winter's day. Tasty and tremendously satisfying, oats are high in fibre and a perfect way to ensure the family is alert and ready for an energised day ahead.

Tinned fish

Making tasty meals is easy when you store tinned sardines, tuna and anchovies in your pantry. Bursting with anti-inflammatory properties, these little guys are budget-friendly and tremendously convenient to keep on hand if you prefer preparing fresh meals swiftly but don't want to sacrifice flavour. When you're strapped for time but keen on eating a balanced meal with adequate protein and good fats, adding a tin of sardines to a salad is a good solution.

Tinned tomatoes

From pasta sauces to vegetable bakes and soups to casseroles, there's no limit to what trusty tinned tomatoes can do for your kitchen, especially if you don't have fresh on hand. They add a richness of flavour to many a meal, and are a versatile product to have on hand. When transforming a roast into a stew, or converting unused vegetables into pasta, tinned tomatoes are essential for simple but flavoursome cooking.

Pulses

Pulses (or legumes) will play a key role in your supercharged kitchen. Stocking chickpeas, cannellini beans, lentils and other pulses is a convenient and inexpensive way to jazz up the left-over vegetables from last night's dinner. Create a lentil curry or chickpea salad in a flash, or make mouth-watering dips.

Pulses provide protein, complex carbohydrates and several vitamins and minerals that give sustained energy throughout the day. They're known to lower blood pressure and reduce LDL cholesterol levels, adding a supercharged kick to any meal.

Unopened raw pulses can last for years in the pantry, reducing the chance of waste, and are really simple to prepare. Once you've cooked up a batch of your favourite pulse, you can store any unused portion in the fridge for up to five days as a quick and easy addition to your remaining week's meals.

Dressings, oils and vinegars

To add some instant flavour and bring your ingredients together, maintain stocks of a few basic dressings, oils and vinegars. Start with wheat-free tamari, apple cider vinegar and extra virgin olive oil. Wheat-free tamari is a thicker, less salty, fermented soy sauce that can be used in Asian and non-Asian cooking to add a full, savoury umami flavour to your dishes.

Originally used as a food preservative, vinegar is a must-have condiment for flavour and acidic balance. Apple cider vinegar, is delicious as a marinade or salad dressing, and is known for its vast list of medicinal benefits, including supporting digestion and providing an energy boost.

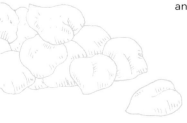

Extra virgin olive oil is a necessity in a supercharged kitchen, and you may find yourself using it daily. The 'extra virgin' refers to the oil being of the highest quality, harvested when the fruit is at its peak and processed straight away. Extra virgin olive oil is completely natural, and it tastes so rich and charming it's no wonder the Italians add it to everything!

Seeds and nuts

These are some of the most adaptable ingredients, adding a crunchy texture and earthy flavour to your sweet or savoury dishes. They also taste great on their own as a nifty little nibble. Keep on hand almonds, hazelnuts, cashews, pecans, walnuts, pine nuts and pistachios.

If you haven't experimented much with seeds, try chia and linseeds (flaxseeds). Sprinkle chia seeds over your breakfast parfait, or simply scatter them over a fruit salad for some added protein and fibre. You can eat linseeds whole – sprinkled over your breakfast or used in home-made muesli bars, say. Another way to use linseeds is in breads and muffins, after grinding them to meal using a high-speed blender (or you can buy them ready-ground at the supermarket).

Nut and seed butters are a scrumptious and filling spread to add to crackers or vegetable sticks. A favourite of mine is tahini, made from ground sesame seeds. My Tarator Sauce (page 310), made with tahini, is delicious poured over an avocado and smoked salmon salad. It's also handy for transforming dishes: added to casseroles, roasted vegetables or even smoothies, tahini lends a thick and creamy texture.

Natural sweeteners

Alternatives to refined sugar and artificial sweeteners include rice malt syrup, raw honey, stevia and fruits. They're a good way to satisfy your sweet tooth while protecting your waistline.

TRY THIS: Squeeze the juice from your favourite citrus fruit into some freshly brewed green tea. Chill, then add some sparkling water, fresh mint and stevia to sweeten. The ultimate iced tea!

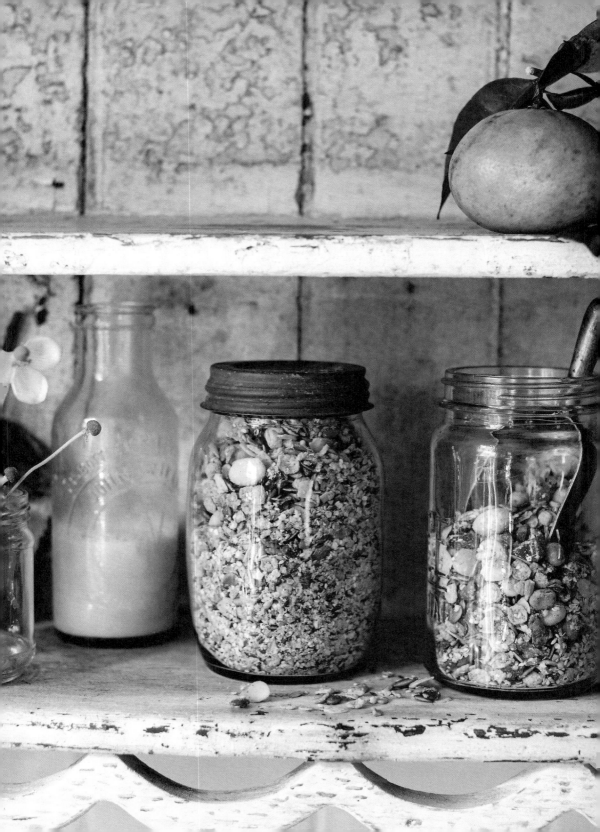

FRIDGE

The fridge is also an important component of any supercharged kitchen. To add an extra hit of flavour and get really creative with your cooking, here are my favourite fridge-friendly foods.

Tomato paste (concentrated purée), pesto and olives

These ingredients are always in my fridge, and I use them on pizzas or pasta, or in dips or winter casseroles. Having these ingredients on hand ensures that when the time comes to transform meals, you're all set to get crafty without any time-wasting. They offer a very convenient opportunity to convert unused vegetables into spiralised pasta with a fresh pesto or marinara sauce in just minutes.

Cheeses and yoghurts

Goat's and sheep's cheeses have some of the most charming flavours and aromas. These are wonderful for crumbling over salads or simply added to a tray with fruit, crackers or vegetable sticks as a satisfying snack. Having cheese on hand allows you to jazz up a salad or a platter of left-over vegetables and meats to add a gourmet touch. If you're dairy-free, you can try my non-dairy Vegan Cheese Platter (page 288).

Moving right along, goat's, sheep's or coconut yoghurts are a delightful addition to your supercharged kitchen. Use them to craft a creamy yet light dressing for a salad or simply enjoy them with some berries and granola scattered on top.

Non-dairy milks

A natural nut milk, oat milk, coconut milk, rice milk or seed milk (hemp!) is a delightful non-dairy option to add to your breakfast muesli or porridge. If you're extra-handy in the kitchen, you can always make your own. When creating curries, soups, casseroles or stews, or even thickening up a sauce or gravy to pour over meat, coconut milk is a close friend.

Purchase non-dairy milks in the carton and store in your pantry until you're ready to use. Once opened, the carton should be stored in the fridge and used within a few days.

FREEZER

Depending on the size of your freezer, some of the essential freezer nitty-gritties to have on hand are home-made stock, and frozen vegies and berries. Other odds and ends that can keep in your freezer are ginger, dough or batter, vegie burgers, edamame (soya bean pods), nuts, flaxseed meal, flours and muffin mixes.

Frozen vegetables

You get home from work hungry and tired, and there are no fresh ingredients in the fridge but you want to eat something right away. Your first thought might be, *What's the number to order in?* The perfect solution is to have a couple of packets of snap-frozen vegetables in your freezer. Stock up on edamame, spinach, broccoli and green beans. They'll come in handy when you need a quick satisfying bite. Then all you need do is open your pantry and add your choice of pulses and tinned tomatoes or a pre-made sauce, and voilà! You have everything you need to create a home-cooked dinner in just minutes.

Frozen berries

A final must-have for your freezer is frozen berries. I know their list of health benefits is as long as your arm, but you'll often find me eating them simply because they taste so sweet and satisfying. Fresh berries are delicious, but if you know you have a busy week and may run the risk of wasting those sweet fruits, keeping frozen berries on hand avoids waste. And they make a convenient solution for an uplifting smoothie or a refreshing breakfast, scattered over a granola or yoghurt. Try mixing frozen berries into your next sweet dessert, or start with my Kakadu Plum and Blueberry Ice Cream (page 54).

Saffron brown rice porridge with apple

{ *SERVES 2* }

Porridge never goes out of fashion because there are so many creative ways to jazz it up and transform your morning from mundane to magic. The flavours of India provided by cinnamon, cardamom and saffron, combined with a swap from traditional oats to nourishing brown rice, will keep you on your toes. This is a beautifully grounding autumnal breakfast, to be enjoyed with a steaming pot of herbal tea. The perfect recipe for a slow-boat Sunday morning.

220 g (7³/₄ oz/1 cup) brown rice, soaked in filtered water for 1 hour and drained

1 litre (35 fl oz/4 cups) coconut or almond milk, plus extra to serve

1 apple, peeled, cored and cut into matchsticks, plus extra to serve

15 g (¹/₂ oz/¹/₄ cup) coconut flakes (optional)

45 g (1¹/₂ oz/¹/₃ cup) pistachio nut kernels, roughly chopped, plus extra to serve

50 g (1³/₄ oz/¹/₃ cup) raw cashews, roughly chopped

8 saffron threads

5 cardamom pods, bruised or crushed

1 teaspoon ground cinnamon

¹/₂ teaspoon alcohol-free vanilla extract or vanilla powder

sea salt, to taste

2 tablespoons raw honey or rice malt syrup, to serve (optional)

dehydrated/roasted apple slices, to serve (optional)

edible flowers, to serve (optional)

Mix the rice and milk in a large saucepan over medium heat and bring to the boil. Add the apple, coconut flakes, if using, nuts, spices and vanilla. Reduce the heat to low and simmer, covered, for 30 minutes, or until all the milk has been absorbed and the rice is cooked through. Season with salt and sweeten, if you like.

Serve topped with extra chopped pistachio nuts, apple matchsticks and milk. Add a dehydrated apple slice and an edible flower or two, if using.

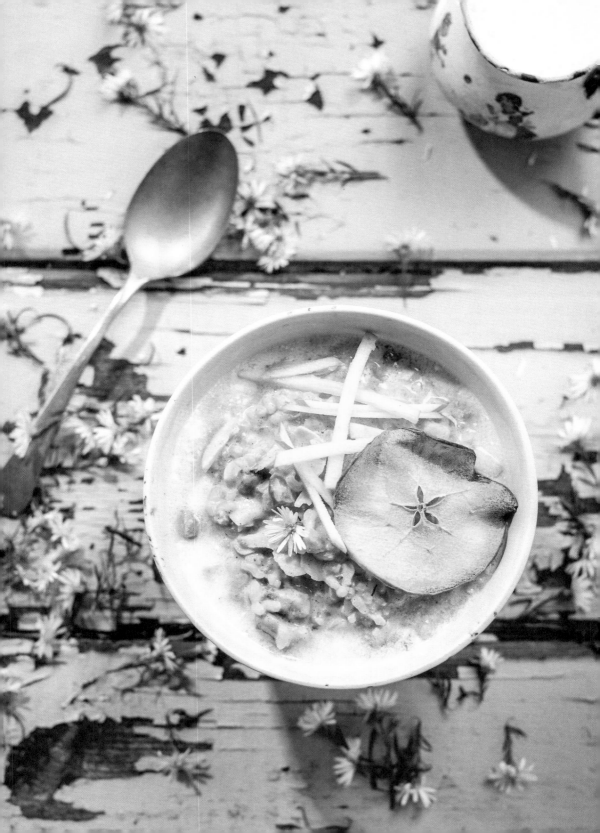

Macadamia, garlic and parsnip soup

{ *SERVES* 2-3 }

3 large parsnips, peeled and cut into 2 cm (³/₄ inch) rounds or dice

10 garlic cloves, sliced

1 large brown onion, roughly chopped

1 tablespoon extra virgin olive oil, plus extra (optional) for drizzling

155 g (5¹/₂ oz/1 cup) macadamia nuts, soaked in warm filtered water for 30 minutes, plus extra (optional), chopped, to serve

1 litre (35 fl oz/4 cups) vegetable stock or filtered water

1 tablespoon apple cider vinegar

1 teaspoon dried thyme

1 teaspoon dried rosemary

sea salt and freshly ground black pepper, to taste

thyme sprigs, to serve

Preheat the oven to 200°C (400°F).

Spread the parsnips, garlic and onion in a roasting tin, add the olive oil and toss to coat. Roast for 25–30 minutes, until the vegetables are tender and lightly browned.

While the vegetables are cooking, drain the soaked macadamias

Transfer the roasted vegetables to a large saucepan and add the macadamias, stock, apple cider vinegar, herbs, salt and pepper. Bring to the boil over medium heat, then reduce the heat to low and simmer, covered, for 10 minutes. Allow to cool slightly, then purée in a food processor or blender until smooth and creamy.

Serve immediately, topped with extra chopped macadamias and a drizzle of extra olive oil, if using, black pepper and thyme sprigs.

SUPERCHARGED TIP

You can make this soup extra delicious by topping with small parsnips sliced lengthways and roasted.

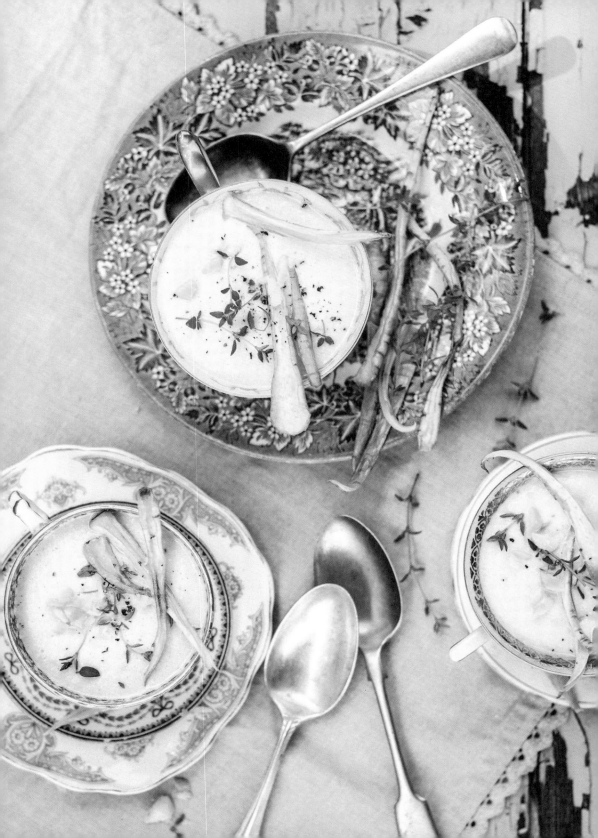

Chicken and brown rice soup with kale and walnuts

{ *SERVES* 2–3 }

2 tablespoons olive oil

1 brown onion, chopped

2 celery stalks, sliced

2 large carrots, chopped

1 red capsicum (pepper),
  seeded and chopped

2 garlic cloves, sliced

60 g (2¼ oz/½ cup) walnuts

500 g (1 lb 2 oz) minced
  (ground) chicken

2 teaspoons mixed dried herbs
  (e.g. basil, sage, rosemary,
  thyme)

350 g (12 oz/1 small bunch) kale,
  stems and spines removed,
  chopped

1 teaspoon sea salt,
  or to taste

½ teaspoon freshly ground
  black pepper, or to taste

1 litre (35 fl oz/4 cups) chicken
  stock, plus extra as needed

2 tablespoons wheat-free
  tamari

1 teaspoon lemon zest

juice of 1 small lemon

400 g (14 oz) tinned diced
  tomatoes

185 g (6½ oz/1 cup) cooked
  brown rice

small handful flat-leaf (Italian)
  parsley, chopped, to serve

Heat the olive oil in a large saucepan over medium–high heat. Add the onion, celery, carrots and capsicum, then cook until the onion is translucent. Add the garlic and walnuts, then cook for a further 2 minutes. Add the chicken and stir until cooked through, about 5 minutes. Stir in the herbs, then add the kale and season with salt and pepper.

Add the stock, tamari, lemon zest and juice, and tomatoes to the saucepan. Bring to the boil, then reduce the heat to medium–low and simmer for 15–20 minutes, until the vegetables are tender.

Towards the end of cooking, stir in the rice and cook until warmed through. Ladle into bowls and serve garnished with the parsley.

Warm green bean salad

{ *SERVES* 4 }

60 ml (2 fl oz/¼ cup) extra
   virgin olive oil

1 large brown onion, diced

2 garlic cloves, sliced

500 g (1 lb 2 oz) green beans,
   trimmed

1 teaspoon ground turmeric

½ teaspoon chilli powder or
   chilli flakes

1½ teaspoons sea salt

20 g (¾ oz/¼ cup) shredded
   coconut, plus extra to serve

Heat the olive oil in a medium saucepan over medium-high heat. Sauté the onion and garlic for 3–4 minutes, until the onion is translucent, then add the green beans. Reduce the heat to low and cook, covered, for 5 minutes. Stir in the remaining ingredients, and cook, stirring, for a further 5 minutes.

Transfer to a bowl to cool a little. Top with extra coconut and serve.

Baked sweet veg mash

{ *SERVES* 4 *AS A SIDE* }

I adore a blend of earthy parsnips, sweet potato and swedes (rutabaga), but encourage you to snap up whatever Mother Nature is offering in your garden or local farmers' market.

600 g (1 lb 5 oz) chopped and
   steamed root vegetables

2 garlic cloves, crushed

pinch of sea salt

freshly ground black pepper,
   to taste

1 tablespoon nut butter
   (optional)

1 tablespoon nutritional yeast
   flakes (optional)

1 tablespoon rice malt syrup

20 g (¾ oz) butter, melted,
   or 1 tablespoon extra virgin
   olive oil

Preheat the oven to 220°C (425°F).

Roughly mash the vegetables, garlic, salt and pepper, nut butter and nutritional yeast flakes, if using, with a fork, or purée in a food processor. Transfer to a square baking dish, scrape across the top with a fork to create little trenches and drizzle over the rice malt syrup and butter.

Bake for 15–20 minutes, until the top is crispy.

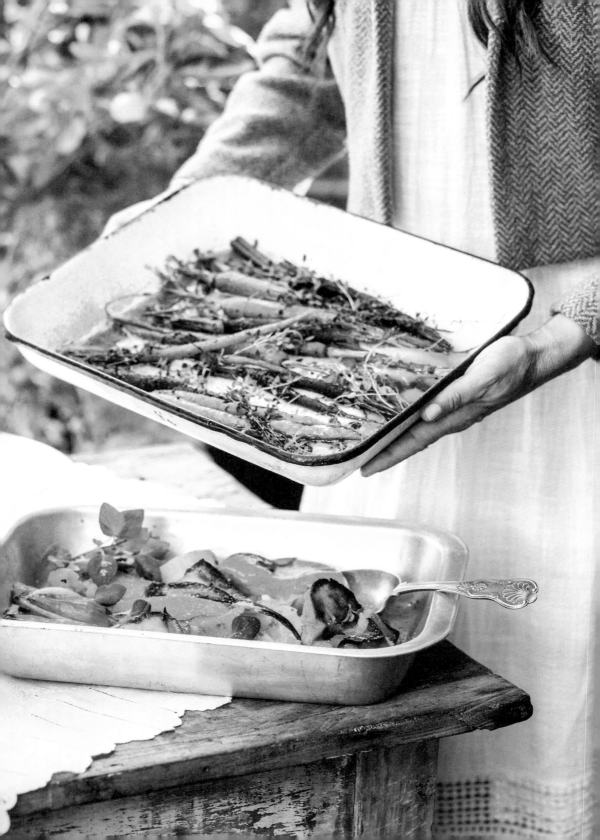

Sweet lemon thyme roasted carrots

{ *SERVES* 2 }

Heirloom carrots are probably one of my favourite sights when gathering seasonal produce. I love their spirally little bottom roots like tendrils, luscious green tops and the remarkable amount of colour they can add to a dish. They're such a treat to roast, and this recipe preserves their full form and flavour, elevating them with caramelised rice malt syrup. This is the perfect accompaniment for roasted meats.

2 tablespoons extra virgin olive oil

90 g (3¼ oz/¼ cup) rice malt syrup

1 tablespoon lemon juice

1 tablespoon apple cider vinegar

6 lemon thyme sprigs

sea salt and freshly ground black pepper, to taste

500 g (1 lb 2 oz) heirloom or baby carrots, peeled and trimmed

Preheat the oven to 200°C (400°F).

Combine all the ingredients except the carrots in a small bowl and stir well.

Spread out the carrots in a large roasting tin, drizzle over the dressing and toss to combine. Roast for 25–30 minutes, until the carrots are cooked through.

One-pan salmon with greens

{ *SERVES* 1 }

I'm so grateful for salmon. It's so clean and pure in flavour, and one of my ideal protein sources, both for its health benefits and its luxuriousness when presented simply. This pan-fried salmon with asparagus, fresh herbs and sweet tomatoes is a lovely, fresh and incredibly easy lunch or dinner. Seek out wild-caught salmon for its superior quality and flavour.

40 g (1½ oz) butter or
2 tablespoons extra virgin
olive oil, plus extra as needed
and for drizzling

1 × 150–180 g (5½–6¼ oz)
salmon fillet or cutlet, skin on

6 large sage leaves

6 asparagus spears, woody
ends trimmed

large handful baby English
spinach leaves

8 small tomatoes, halved if
large

handful mint leaves

sea salt, to taste

½ lemon (optional)

Heat the butter in a medium frying pan over medium heat. Add the salmon, skin side down for a fillet, and the sage leaves, then cook for 3–4 minutes. Turn the salmon over, add the asparagus, and fry the other side for 2 minutes, or until cooked to your liking. Remove the sage from the pan once it's crispy and the asparagus when cooked through, with brown patches but not burnt. Add the spinach and tomatoes to the pan with a little extra butter if needed (but there should be enough pan juices).

Meanwhile, tear the mint leaves and spread them on a plate. Top with the tomatoes, drizzle over a little olive oil and season with salt.

Add the salmon, spinach and asparagus, and squeeze lemon juice over the top, if using. Garnish with the fried sage leaves.

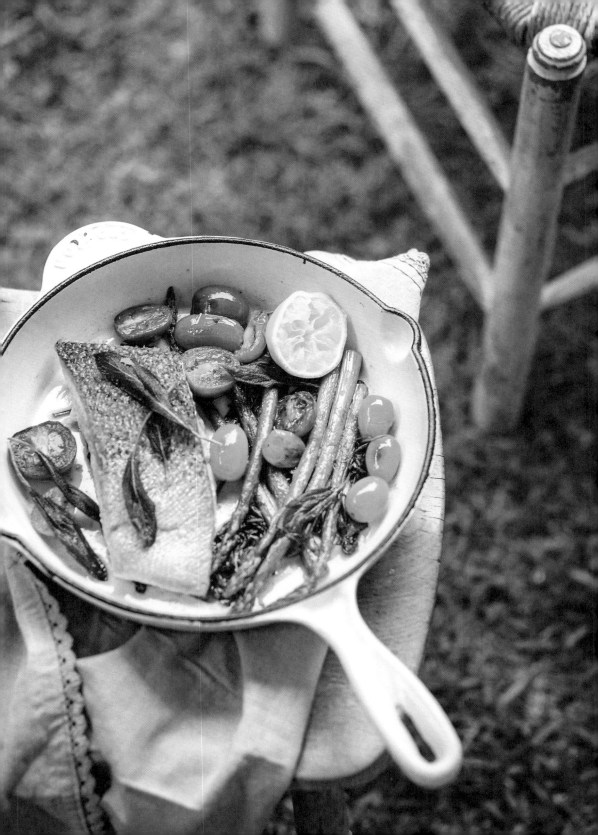

Easy-peasy minted peas with goat's cheese and bacon

{ *SERVES* 4 }

Bacon. The sad reason why I could never be a full vegetarian. I just delight in the scent of grilling bacon far too much. And its ability to add ridiculous amounts of flavour to a dish continues to astound me. It's worth investing in high-quality organic or free-range nitrate-free bacon to bring flavour to a range of dishes from omelettes to soups, or as a vital element in these scrummy minted peas alongside melt-in-your-mouth creamy goat's cheese.

420 g (14³/₄ oz/3 cups) frozen peas

4 nitrate-free bacon rashers (slices)

150 g (5¹/₂ oz) goat's cheese, diced

handful mint leaves, finely chopped

sea salt and freshly ground black pepper, to taste

handful coriander (cilantro) leaves, chopped

Heat the grill (broiler) to medium.

Warm the peas in a medium saucepan over low heat.

Meanwhile, grill the bacon then chop roughly.

Add the bacon, cheese and mint to the peas, and cook until the cheese is slightly melted. Season with salt and pepper. Serve topped with the coriander.

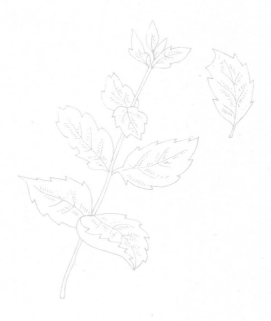

Savoury mince

{ *SERVES* 3 }

Mince (ground meat) is an economical and delicious staple in my household that forms the basis of so many meals. This savoury mince is an excellent recipe to cook in batches using your favourite meat – triple the quantities and store portions in your freezer for stuffing roasted capsicums (peppers) or butternut pumpkin (squash), layering in a lasagne, or as the basis for a bolognese. I love to eat this alongside a serving of Baked Sweet Veg Mash (see page 91), or to scatter it over salads as a larb (Lao meat salad) for deep-flavoured protein meal.

2 teaspoons ghee

80 g (2¾ oz/½ cup) finely chopped onion

3–5 large garlic cloves, crushed

1 × 2.5 cm (1 inch) piece fresh ginger, grated or very thinly sliced

1 hot green chilli, very thinly sliced, seeds removed

500 g (1 lb 2 oz) minced (ground) meat

2 teaspoons lemon juice

handful mint leaves, finely chopped

½ teaspoon cumin seeds, roughly crushed

1 teaspoon red chilli flakes (optional)

sea salt and freshly ground black pepper, to taste

cooked brown rice and pre-packaged dried coconut chutney (optional), to serve

Heat the ghee in a large heavy-based frying pan over medium heat, then sauté the onion and garlic for 3–4 minutes, until the onion is translucent. Add the ginger and fresh chilli, then cook for a further 2 minutes. Add the meat and stir until cooked through, then add the lemon juice, mint, spices, salt and pepper.

Serve on brown rice and top with dried coconut chutney, if using.

Beef stir-fry with peaches

{ *SERVES* 3-4 }

1 tablespoon sesame oil or
  coconut oil

300 g (10½ oz) beef rump or
  sirloin, cut into strips

3 garlic cloves, crushed

1 × 5 cm (2 inch) piece fresh
  ginger, grated

4 peaches or nectarines,
  halved, stone removed and
  cut into wedges

800 g (1 lb 12 oz/2 small
  bunches) bok choy (pak choy)

1 tablespoon coconut aminos or
  wheat-free tamari

2 tablespoons rice malt syrup

Cauliflower Rice (page 166),
  to serve

Heat the sesame oil in a wok over medium-high heat and stir-fry the beef strips until browned, working in batches if necessary. Add the garlic and ginger, and stir-fry for 1 minute. Add the peaches and cook for 3 minutes, or until caramelised. Transfer to a bowl and set aside.

Return the wok to the heat, add the bok choy and aminos, and stir until the bok choy has wilted. Add the rice malt syrup and return the beef and peaches to the wok, stirring gently to warm through.

Serve with the cauliflower rice.

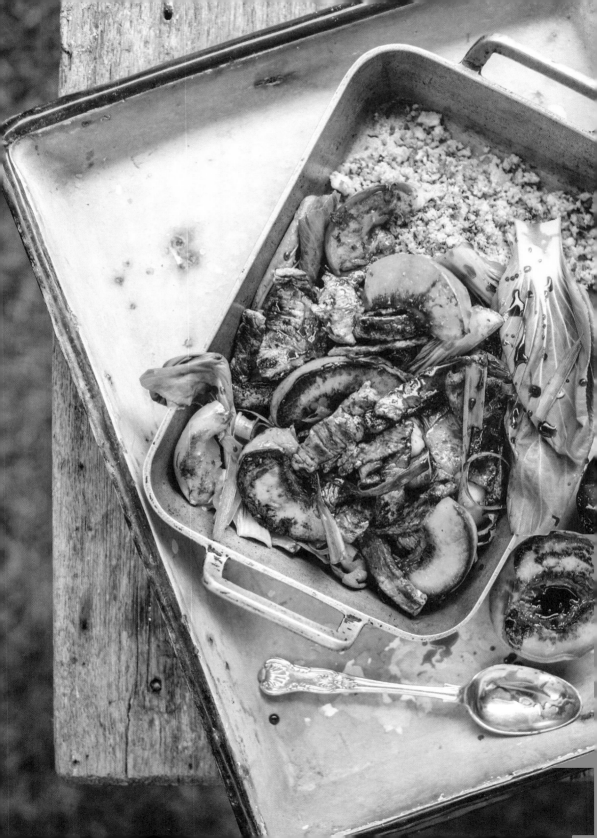

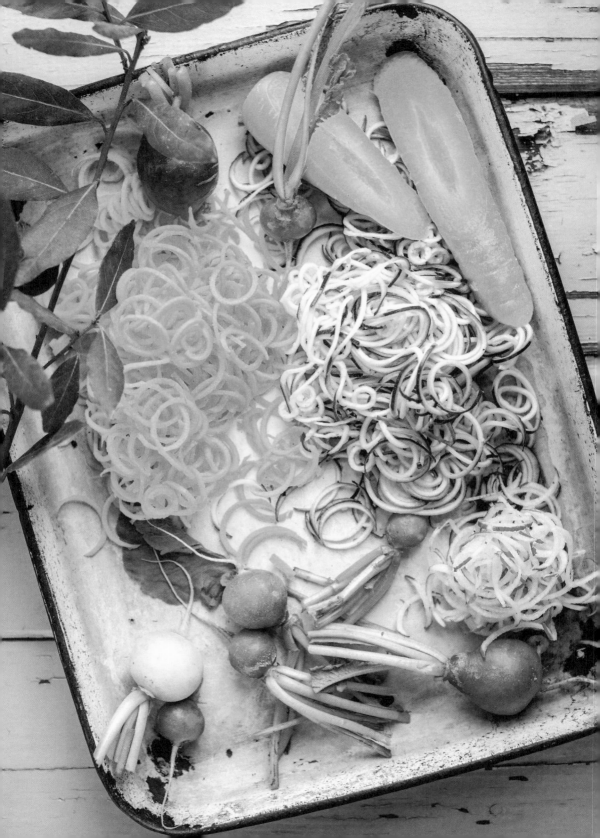

Simplifying meal preparation

Remember that purposeful and fulfilling eating is possible even if you're short of time and feeding a big family or if you're a cash-strapped student.

First and foremost, when starting out, don't try to do so much that you're feeling overwhelmed. Just begin slowly by including more fresh ingredients, but don't be restrictive. As you become more comfortable with using whole foods, try to include as many colours as possible in your dishes – you're aiming to eat the rainbow so that you can fill your body with a variety of nutrients. Diversity is the key!

If preparation is where you feel most challenged, clear off the work surface and get ready for some fun and interesting meal-prep ideas:

- Chop up or spiralise raw vegetables such as carrots, celery, zucchini (courgettes) and capsicums (peppers) into strips, batons and sticks, and store in the fridge. Then all you need do is whip up a quick dip for a delicious snack.

- When roasting batches of vegetables on high heat to bring out their sweetness, find perfect partners with the same cooking times. Fast-cooking vegetables are asparagus, capsicum, broccoli, leeks, mushrooms, tomatoes and zucchini, while slow-roasting vegetables include celeriac, parsnips, potatoes, carrots, cauliflower, swede (rutabaga), daikon (mooli), butternut pumpkin (squash) and onions. If you require a mixture of fast and slow, cook slower vegetables on the stovetop first and then add to the baking dish. For a handy guide to the art of cooking vegetables, see page 104.

- Smoothies can be made in advance and frozen in muffin trays. When morning comes, take three out and simply whiz them in a high-speed blender.

- When cooking something like chicken, cook two at the same time but with a couple of variations. One could be lemon and rosemary and the other Moroccan spices with yoghurt.

- Eggs can be hard-boiled in muffin trays in the oven allowing you to cook a few batches of 12 at a time and store them to add quickly to salads for extra protein. Simply preheat the oven to 175°C (345°F), place a whole egg (in its shell) in each muffin hole, no water, and bake for 30 minutes. Cool in iced water if you need to peel them immediately.

- Make a batch of frittatas in muffin trays, which can be stored in the fridge for up to five days. You won't lose interest if you make them in different flavours.

- Pre-assemble glass jars of soup ingredients; salads; or layered gluten-free oatmeal, buckwheat, coconut milk and berries. Glass jars help prevent the ingredients spoiling. Carry dressings separately, or place them at the bottom of the jar, under a layer of sturdier vegetables such as capsicum and carrots, then top with leafy greens. A wad of paper towel at the top will absorb moisture and enable you to store your soups and salad jars for three to five days.

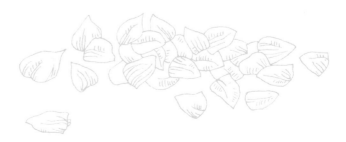

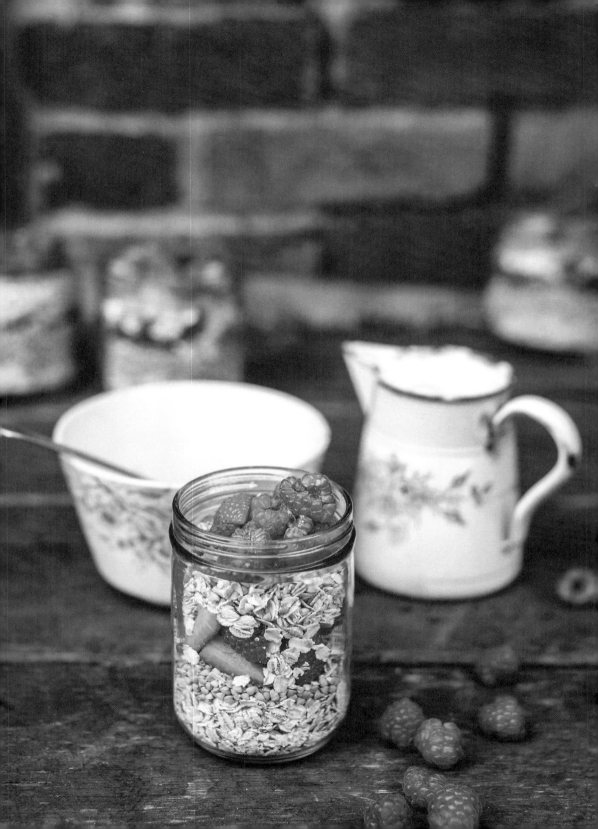

The art of cooking vegetables

Just because vegetables are good for us doesn't mean they need to be portrayed as a moustache-twirling dastardly villain! Or that eating them should be seen as an unfortunate yet necessary chore.

While some of us, particularly children, will cross the street to avoid vegetables, they really are the gift that keeps on giving. The secret to eating more vegetables is to prepare them in a way that makes them just as delicious as the foods they're partnered with. In fact, vegetables can be the flavour hero of the show if you know how to bring out their trademark charm.

While it may seem strange, cooking vegetables is a skill that not everyone has mastered – press rewind and take a look at your last aeroplane or takeaway meal. Okay, case closed. The most important thing to remember when cooking vegetables is that each one needs to be treated as an individual, just like any leading act. Some, such as onions, are better sautéed, while others, like root vegetables, are delicious roasted, to draw out their natural sweetness. A variety of leafy greens are best served steamed, while other vegies simply taste better raw.

Each cooking method has its advantages and disadvantages, and each gives different vegetables a particular flavour and texture. Always remember to wash your vegetables thoroughly before preparation, regardless of whether they're organic. Buying vegetables from farmers' markets rather than large supermarket chains will give you fresher produce and access to a range of varieties that the supermarkets don't carry.

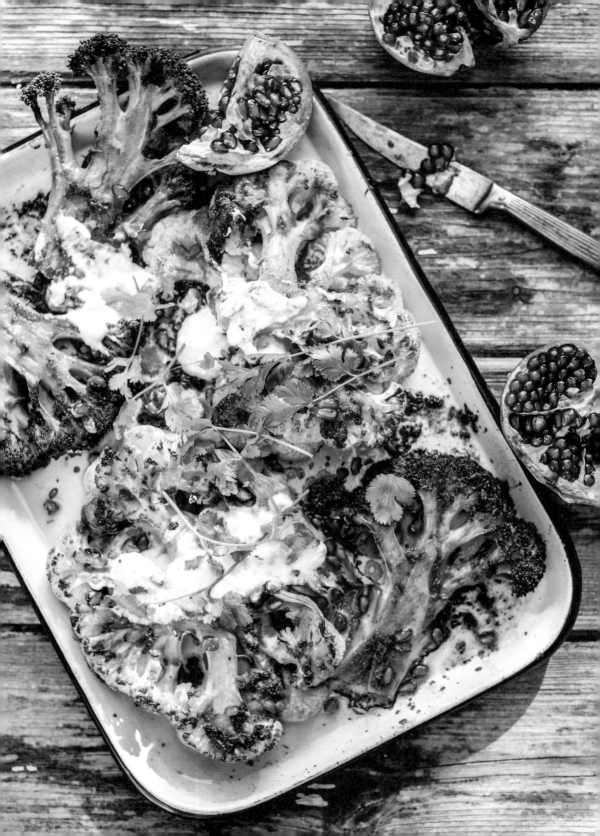

BOILING

While boiling is one of the quickest and most convenient ways to prepare vegetables – exhibit A: one cooking pot; exhibit B: enough water to cover – it's my least recommended method. The boiling water can draw flavour and nutrients out of the vegetables, leaving them bland and watery, and robbing you of their nutritional powers.

If boiling vegetables is your only option, minimise nutrient and flavour loss by ensuring they spend minimal time in the boiling water. You can allow the vegetables to cook faster by chopping them into very small even chunks, just before boiling so they remain fresh. Bring the water to the boil before adding the vegetables. For green leafy vegetables, use as much water as possible, so the vegetables don't cool down the water, while all other vegetables should be boiled in as little water as possible to reduce nutrient loss. The best way to test whether your vegetables are cooked is to try the largest piece, being careful not to burn yourself.

You'll have your personal preference as to how crisp you like your vegetables. I like al dente – cooking veg to a pulpy mess is enough to give anyone the creeps.

STEAMING

A method frequently employed in Asian cultures, steaming is a dependable alternative to boiling, as it cooks and softens vegetables without them losing as many nutrients, given they are never actually immersed in the water. Steaming is also an incredibly healthy way to prepare your vegetables, as it requires no oils.

While you can purchase fancy steaming appliances, all you really need is a pot of boiling water and a steaming basket, which can be purchased cheaply from most Asian grocers or discount stores. You can even use a colander if you have one handy.

Prepare the vegetables in the same way you would to boil them, then place them in the steaming basket (or colander) over a pot with 5–10 cm (2–4 inches) deep boiling water. Cover the steaming basket and in a few minutes your vegies are done. Just be careful not to absent-mindedly lean over the steaming basket when removing the lid, as steam burns can be a real fly in the ointment when it comes to enjoying your freshly made veg. No fair! Also be sure to check the water level frequently – you don't want it to run out or you'll end up in a cloud of smoke.

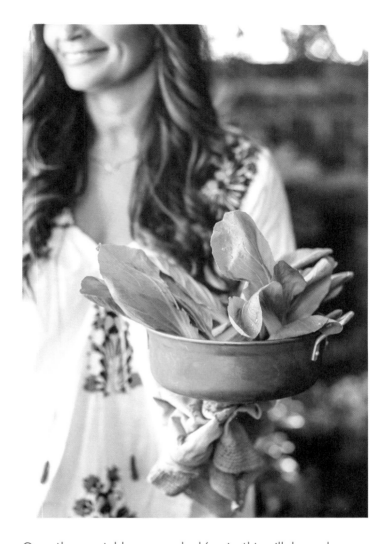

Once the vegetables are cooked (again, this will depend on personal preference, but see pages 108–109 for some guidance), you can either serve them like this or make a combo by adding a little seasoning, a healthy oil such as olive or flaxseed, herbs, spices, citrus juices, nuts and seeds, or a sauce such as tamari. No need to swamp them in pesky processed sauces – a supercharged kitchen uses real ingredients.

Other vegetables that can be steamed are capsicums (peppers) and garlic, but it's worth mentioning that they may be better suited to roasting, to retain their texture and bring out their unique flavours.

STEAMING VEGETABLES

VEGETABLE	SIZE AND PREPARATION	STEAMING TIME
ARTICHOKES	Whole	30–50 minutes
ASPARAGUS	Whole thick spears	8–10 minutes
	Cut into 5 cm (2 inch) lengths	4–7 minutes
BEANS, GREEN	Whole	5–15 minutes
BEETROOT (BEETS)	Whole, unpeeled, scrubbed clean (remove the skin after steaming)	40–50 minutes
BROCCOLI	Halved florets	5–8 minutes
BRUSSELS SPROUTS	Trimmed and halved	6–12 minutes
BUTTERNUT PUMPKIN (SQUASH)	Peeled and cut into 2 cm (¾ inch) cubes	7–10 minutes
CABBAGE	Roughly sliced	5–8 minutes
	Cut into wedges	6–9 minutes
CARROTS	Cut into 2 cm (¾ inch) slices	5–7 minutes
	Whole baby	10–15 minutes
CAULIFLOWER	Whole	10–15 minutes
	Quartered florets	6–10 minutes
CELERY	Cut into 2 cm (¾ inch) slices	4–9 minutes
EGGPLANT (AUBERGINE)	Whole	15–30 minutes
	Cut into 2 cm (¾ inch) cubes	5–6 minutes

VEGETABLE	SIZE AND PREPARATION	STEAMING TIME
FENNEL	Cut crossways into 2 cm (¾ inch) slices	8–10 minutes
KALE	Spines removed	4–7 minutes
KOHLRABI	Whole	30–35 minutes
LEEKS	Pale part only, trimmed and halved	5–8 minutes
MUSHROOMS	Whole	4–5 minutes
ONIONS	Whole, peeled	8–12 minutes
PARSNIPS	Peeled and cut into 2 cm (¾ inch) slices	8–10 minutes
PEAS	Fresh, shelled	2–4 minutes
POTATOES	Peeled or scrubbed clean and cut into 2 cm (¾ inch) cubes	10–12 minutes
RADISHES	Whole, trimmed	7–14 minutes
SPINACH	Stalks trimmed off	5–6 minutes
SUGARSNAP PEAS	Whole pods, trimmed	5–6 minutes
SWEET POTATOES	Cut into 2 cm (¾ inch) cubes	8–12 minutes
TOMATOES	Whole	2–3 minutes
TURNIPS	Cut into 2 cm (¾ inch) cubes	10–12 minutes
ZUCCHINI (COURGETTES)	Cut into 5 cm (2 inch) slices	5–10 minutes

SAUTÉING AND STIR-FRYING

Sautéing or stir-frying vegetables involves cooking them in oil in a frying pan, wok or saucepan over high heat and stirring them often. In fact, the word *sauté* comes from the French for 'jump'. The high heat means vegetables cook quickly, minimising nutrient loss, while the frequent stirring ensures they don't burn or stick to the pan.

This method can be used if you want a slightly crisp texture. It's more involved than boiling or steaming, but it's a great option because the vegetables retain much more flavour. Better yet, when combined with a bit of heat-resistant oil (such as coconut oil), spices and/or a marinade, sautéed vegetables can convert even the most staunchly anti-veg family member.

When choosing a pan to use, try to pick a large one that can hold all your vegies in a single layer and one that's relatively shallow, so the vegetables can be cooked evenly and any steam can escape. To sauté vegetables, heat some oil in the pan over medium to high heat. Add the chopped vegetables, preferably starting with them all at roughly the same room temperature. Stir them frequently until they're nicely browned and cooked through. Season to taste and serve quickly.

Liberal use of spices is the mark of a considerate cook. Ensure you add them just before the end of the sautéing process so they have a little time to warm slightly and release their fragrance and flavour. Fresh herbs can be added after cooking or towards the end. Now here's another warning: if you're adding cheeses or sauces to your vegies, add them in closer towards the end so they don't overcook or burn.

The best vegetables to sauté are cabbage, carrots, onions, corn, asparagus tips, baby artichokes, capsicums (peppers), mushrooms, sugarsnap peas, zucchini (courgettes) and leeks.

Note: You can sauté many more vegetables, but those listed in the table produce the best results.

SAUTÉING OR STIR-FRYING VEGETABLES

VEGETABLE	SIZE AND PREPARATION	SAUTÉING TIME
ARTICHOKES	Hearts	10 minutes
ASPARAGUS	Whole thick spears	4–5 minutes
	Cut into 5 cm (2 inch) pieces	3–4 minutes
BEANS, GREEN	Whole, trimmed	3–4 minutes
BROCCOLI	Small florets	3–4 minutes
BRUSSELS SPROUTS	Trimmed and halved	3–4 minutes
CABBAGE	Shredded	3–4 minutes
CAPSICUMS (PEPPERS)	Sliced into wedges	2–3 minutes
CARROTS	Cut into 2 cm (¾ inch) slices	3–4 minutes
CAULIFLOWER	Small florets	3–4 minutes
CELERY	Cut into 2 cm (¾ inch) slices	3 minutes
CORN	Kernels cut from cob	3 minutes
KALE	Stalks trimmed off	2–3 minutes
LEEKS	White part only, trimmed, cut into 2 cm (¾ inch) slices	2 minutes
MUSHROOMS	Sliced	3 minutes
ONIONS	Peeled and diced	2–3 minutes
PEAS	Fresh, shelled	2–3 minutes
PUMPKIN (SQUASH)	Cut into 2 cm (¾ inch) cubes	3–4 minutes
SPINACH	Spines removed	3 minutes
SUGARSNAP PEAS	Whole pods, trimmed	3–4 minutes
SWEET POTATO	Cut into 2 cm (¾ inch) cubes	3–4 minutes
TURNIPS	Cut into 2 cm (¾ inch) cubes	3–4 minutes
ZUCCHINI (COURGETTES)	Cut into 2 cm (¾ inch) slices	3 minutes

ROASTING

Roasting is my favourite way to prepare vegetables. Softer and moister vegies such as capsicums (peppers), zucchini (courgettes) and asparagus will have much shorter roasting times than hard root vegetables such as parsnips, potatoes and beetroot (beets). Combining vegies with similar roasting times is an easy way to work around this. You can also combine foods with different roasting times by adding the faster-cooking vegetables to the oven later, or by cutting the longer-roasting vegies into much smaller pieces than the softer ones.

To roast vegetables, preheat the oven for about 10 minutes and either line a roasting tin with baking paper or grease it lightly with some of your favourite oil. The first rule about roasting at high heat is you don't talk about roasting with vegetable oils other than coconut oil, which is unique in that it won't oxidise at higher temperatures. If I'm medium- to slow-cooking, I also use olive oil.

If you're roasting without oil, you might like to moisten the vegies by adding a small amount of water, vegetable stock, tomato juice, freshly squeezed lemon or orange juice, tamari or chicken broth to the tin before roasting. (As an aside, when I'm roasting lamb, I often add 80 ml/2½ fl oz/⅓ cup lemon juice to keep it succulent and moist. I sometimes add coconut water too.)

Place the tin on the middle shelf of the oven and check on the vegies frequently, stirring them to ensure they don't stick or burn. Remove them once they're all tender and lightly browned.

ROASTING VEGETABLES*

ROASTING TIME	VEGETABLES
10–15 MINUTES (SHORTER)	asparagus, baby (patty pan) squash, broccoli, capsicum (pepper), cherry tomatoes, garlic, leeks, zucchini (courgettes)
15–20 MINUTES (MODERATE)	brussels sprouts, French shallots, green beans, mushrooms, parsnips, tomatoes
20–30 MINUTES (MEDIUM)	baby artichokes, carrots, eggplant (aubergine), fennel, onions, sweet potato, turnips, swedes (rutabaga)
30–40 MINUTES (LONGER)	celeriac, potatoes
50 MINUTES (LONGEST)	beetroot (beets), pumpkin (winter squash)

* Roasting times are based on the preparation methods specified opposite, in a conventional 230°C (450°F) oven.

FINDING YOUR STYLE

I urge you to go forth and experiment with different vegetable preparation methods to find which ones best suit your lifestyle and taste preferences. Many Western meals (e.g. pastas, casseroles) call for roasted vegetables, while many Asian-style meals involve steaming or stir-frying.

Discover your cooking style, and mix and match methods depending on the occasion and your needs. Don't be afraid to step out of your comfort zone and embrace new techniques or approaches. Your choices are endless, and you may even surprise yourself with what you come up with.

Now is a great time to flip over to the home-grown vegetable section of the book (page 207) and create a list of what you'll be growing, then come back here to learn the powerful potential that resides within a home cook's headquarters, and how to instil your own magic in your supercharged kitchen.

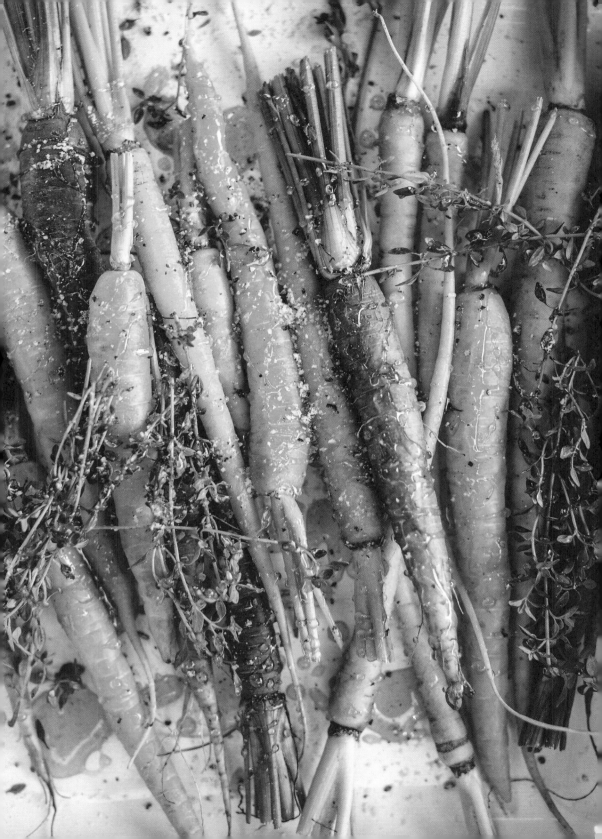

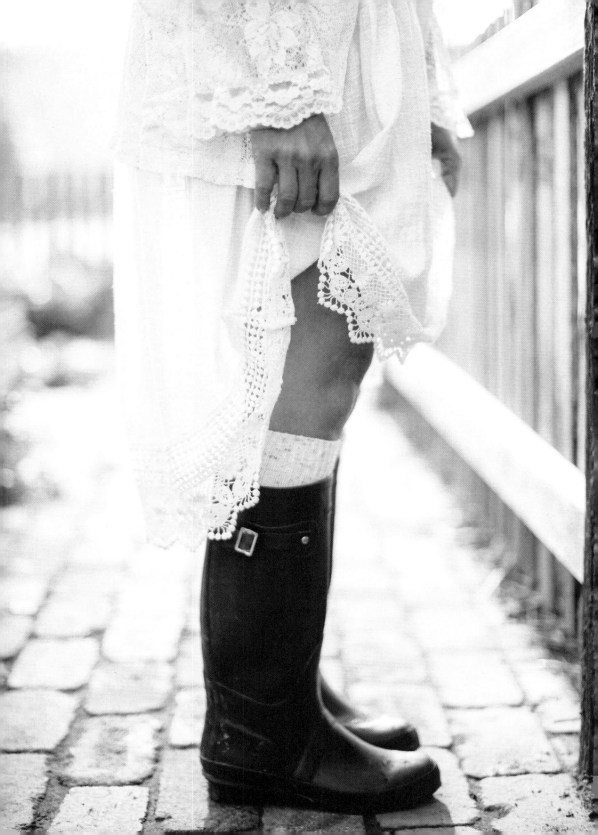

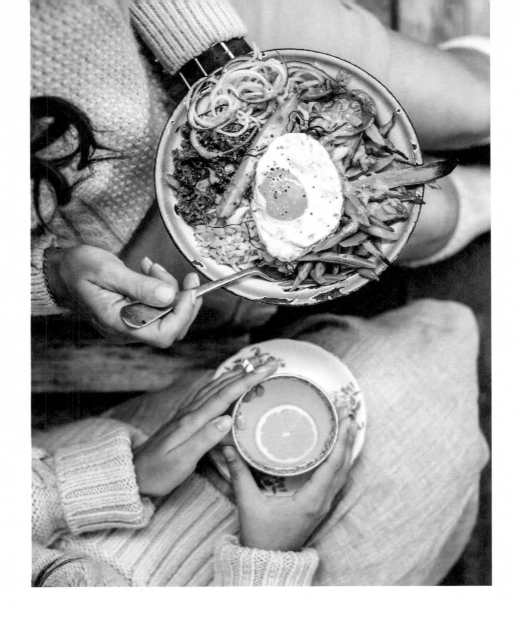

Nourishing breakfast bowl

{ *SERVES 2* }

This is the king of breakfast bowls, and you'll feel like royalty sitting down to this collection of vibrant ingredients first thing in the morning. Loaded with greens, wholesome brown rice, gorgeous orange sweet potato, satiating eggs and a super-tasty tahini-based dressing, this is a great recipe for preparing food mindfully and honouring yourself.

1 sweet potato, peeled and sliced thinly lengthways

2 tablespoons coconut oil, melted, plus extra as needed

sea salt and freshly ground black pepper, to taste

2 heaped tablespoons blanched almonds

2 garlic cloves, chopped

2 spring onions (scallions), chopped

250 g (9 oz/2 cups) sliced green beans

450 g (1 lb/1 bunch) kale, stems and spines removed, roughly chopped

handful baby English spinach leaves

2 eggs

370 g (13 oz/2 cups) hot cooked brown rice

1/2 telegraph (long) cucumber, spiralised into noodles

1 avocado, peeled and sliced

2 sheets nori, torn, or handful dried nori strips

toasted sesame seeds, for sprinkling (optional)

Dressing

65 g (2¼ oz/¼ cup) tahini

60 ml (2 fl oz/¼ cup) filtered water

60 ml (2 fl oz/¼ cup) lemon juice

grated zest of 1 lemon

few drops liquid stevia or your sweetener of choice

1½ teaspoons wheat-free tamari or coconut aminos

½ teaspoon ground turmeric

¼ teaspoon ground ginger

To make the dressing, combine all the ingredients in a jar, seal tightly and shake until combined.

Preheat the oven to 220°C (425°F).

Place the sweet potato in a roasting tin, drizzle over half the coconut oil and bake for 10–15 minutes, until cooked. Season with salt and pepper.

Toast the almonds in a dry frying pan over medium heat and set aside.

Heat the remaining coconut oil in a frying pan over medium heat and sauté the garlic and spring onions for 1–2 minutes. Add the beans and kale, and stir-fry for 3–4 minutes, until cooked through. Add the spinach and cook for 1–2 minutes, until wilted. Move the greens to one side of the pan and fry the eggs to your liking, adding a little more oil if needed.

In two wide shallow bowls, arrange the brown rice, spiralised cucumber, cooked greens and avocado, then top with the almonds, sweet potato, nori and a fried egg. Drizzle the dressing over and sprinkle with sesame seeds, if using, and pepper.

Breakfast hash stack

{ *SERVES* 4 }

350 g (12 oz) small tomatoes, halved if large

olive oil, for drizzling

sea salt and freshly ground black pepper, to taste

handful sage or basil leaves

4 nitrate-free bacon rashers (slices)

butter or olive oil, for frying

8 eggs, whisked

1 tablespoon grated lemon zest

150 g (5½ oz) hard goat's cheese, shaved or soft goat's cheese, crumbled

chopped fresh herbs, to serve

Sweet potato hash brown

4 sweet potatoes, peeled and grated

2 eggs, whisked, plus 1 egg, extra, lightly beaten, for brushing

2 garlic cloves, chopped

1 brown onion, thinly sliced

50 g (1¾ oz/½ cup) almond meal

2 teaspoons sea salt

pinch of freshly grated nutmeg

55 g (2 oz/¼ cup) coconut oil

Preheat the oven to 220°C (425°F).

Put the tomatoes on a baking tray or in an ovenproof frying pan, drizzle over olive oil, season with sea salt and scatter over the sage or basil. Set aside.

To make the hash brown, mix all the ingredients except the coconut oil and extra egg in a bowl. Heat the coconut oil in a frying pan over medium heat, spoon the entire sweet potato mixture into the pan and stir until cooked through. Add to the tomatoes and brush with the extra egg.

Bake the tomatoes and hash brown (see tip) for 10–15 minutes, until the hash brown is crispy. Cut into portions.

Meanwhile, fry the bacon until crispy.

Heat some butter or olive oil in a saucepan over medium–low heat. Add the eggs and move them around the pan with a spatula so they don't stick to the bottom. Add the lemon zest, and cook until just set.

Lay one or two hash brown pieces on each plate, then top with roasted tomatoes, crispy bacon, scrambled egg, goat's cheese and fresh herbs. Season to taste and serve immediately.

SUPERCHARGED TIP

The hash brown can be made ahead of time and frozen for convenience.

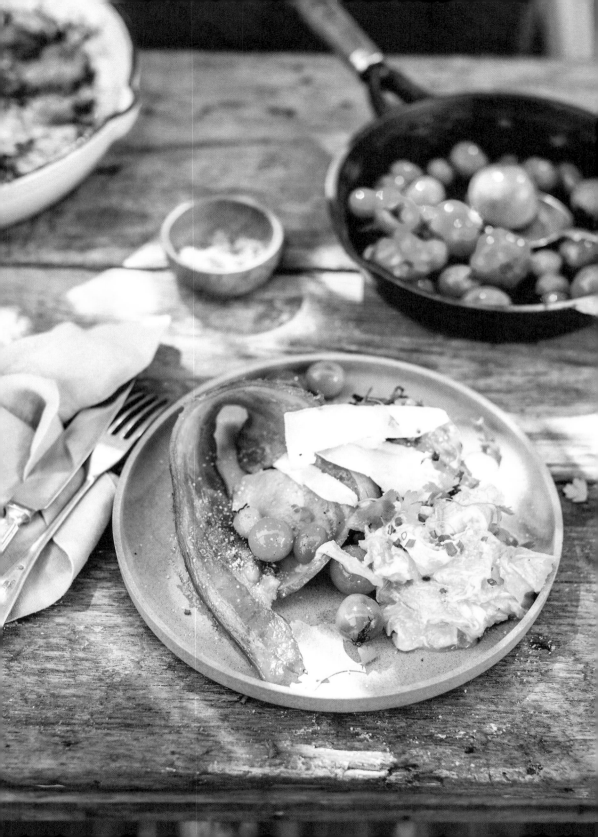

Cumin-spiced lotus root chips

{ *SERVES* 3-4 }

300 g (10½ oz) fresh lotus root
(see tip), peeled and sliced
paper-thin

1 tablespoon avocado oil

1 teaspoon ground cumin

sea salt, to taste

Preheat the oven to 180°C (350°F) and line
a baking tray with baking paper.

In a medium bowl, toss the lotus root with the
avocado oil and cumin until well coated.

Spread out on the prepared baking tray and
bake for 10–12 minutes, until golden brown
and crisp. Season with salt then turn out onto
a wire rack to cool completely – they'll harden
up as they cool.

Note: For a photo of these chips, see
pages 334–35.

SUPERCHARGED TIP
Lotus root is available fresh in Asian
supermarkets and some grocery stores.

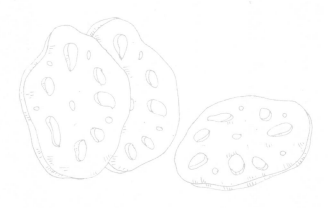

Asparagus, fennel and spinach soup with toasted pepitas

{ *SERVES* 2-3 }

I love finding new ways to experiment with less-common ingredients. Fennel and asparagus are two vegetables that deserve their show-stopping reputation. This soup combines their flavours beautifully and is a unique affair that will linger hours after consumption. The crunchy pepitas, cheesy nutritional yeast flakes and fresh herbs on top offer a special little adornment that will heighten your joy-factor while embellishing a lovely light lunch.

2 tablespoons coconut oil

1 fennel bulb, finely chopped

4 spring onions (scallions), chopped

2 garlic cloves, sliced

450 g (1 lb) asparagus spears, woody ends trimmed, sliced on the diagonal into 2.5 cm (1 inch) lengths

90 g (3¼ oz/2 cups) baby English spinach leaves

750 ml (26 fl oz/3 cups) vegetable stock

1 tablespoon apple cider vinegar

1 teaspoon grated lemon zest

1 tablespoon lemon juice

1 teaspoon ground cumin

sea salt and freshly ground black pepper, to taste

270 ml (9½ fl oz) coconut milk (optional)

2 tablespoons nutritional yeast flakes

75 g (2¾ oz/½ cup) toasted pepitas (pumpkin seeds)

mint and basil leaves, to serve

Heat the coconut oil in a large saucepan over medium heat, then add the fennel, spring onions and garlic, and cook for 2-3 minutes, until softened. Add the asparagus, spinach, stock, vinegar, lemon zest and juice, cumin, salt and pepper. Bring to the boil, then reduce the heat to low and simmer, covered, for 20 minutes. Allow to cool slightly, then transfer to a blender, add the coconut milk and blend until smooth. Return to the pan to warm through.

Ladle into bowls and top with nutritional yeast flakes, pepitas and fresh herbs.

Note: For a photo of this soup, see pages 334-35.

SUPERCHARGED TIP

Roasted asparagus spears and Lotus Root Chips (opposite) make a great garnish, and this soup is delicious with a swirl of Coconut 'Yoghurt' (page 195).

Roasted zucchini and garlic bisque

{ *SERVES* 2 }

1 brown onion, peeled and cut into quarters

1 green capsicum (pepper), cut into quarters, seeded and membranes removed

1 garlic bulb, top sliced off

5 zucchini (courgettes), diced

1 tablespoon coconut oil

small handful basil leaves

½ teaspoon dried oregano

80 g (2¾ oz/½ cup) raw cashews, soaked in filtered water for 2 hours

500 ml (17 fl oz/2 cups) vegetable stock

125 ml (4 fl oz/½ cup) coconut milk

sea salt and freshly ground black pepper, to taste

extra virgin olive oil, for drizzling (optional)

Preheat the oven to 190°C (375°F).

Spread out the onion, capsicum, garlic and zucchini in a roasting tin and brush with the coconut oil. Roast for 25–30 minutes, until cooked through and browned. Remove from the oven and allow to cool, then peel the capsicum and squeeze the garlic cloves from their skins.

Transfer the roasted vegetables to a blender, add the basil, oregano, cashews, stock and coconut milk, and blend until smooth.

Pour into a saucepan, season with salt and pepper, and warm through over medium heat. Serve drizzled with olive oil, if using.

Kaleslaw with creamy sesame dressing

{ SERVES 6 AS A SIDE }

Slaw

4 cups thinly sliced cavolo nero (Tuscan kale)

2 apples, cut into very thin wedges

½ cabbage, thinly sliced

1 red capsicum (pepper), seeded and thinly sliced (optional)

1 small carrot (optional), grated

parsley or microherbs, to serve

Creamy sesame dressing

120 g (4¼ oz/¾ cup) raw cashews, soaked in filtered water for 2 hours

40 g (1½ oz/¼ cup) sesame seeds

50 ml (1¾ fl oz) apple cider vinegar

2 tablespoons sugar-free mustard

1 tablespoon lemon juice

¼ teaspoon sea salt

To make the dressing, pulse all the ingredients in a food processor with a generous splash of filtered water until smooth.

Toss all the slaw ingredients except the herbs in a large bowl and stir through the dressing. Scatter over the herbs, and serve.

Swiss chard with apple cider vinegar

{ *SERVES* 3-4 }

1 kg (2 lb 4 oz/1 bunch) Swiss chard (silverbeet)

50 g (1¾ oz/⅓ cup) pine nuts

2 tablespoons extra virgin olive oil

2 tablespoons sliced French shallots

2 garlic cloves, crushed

60 ml (2 fl oz/¼ cup) apple cider vinegar

sea salt and freshly ground black pepper, to taste

Strip the Swiss chard leaves off the stems and ribs, wash thoroughly and slice thinly.

Heat a large deep frying pan over medium-low heat. Toast the pine nuts, stirring frequently, for 5-7 minutes, until golden brown. Transfer to a bowl and set aside.

Heat the olive oil in the same pan over medium heat and sauté the shallots for 2-3 minutes, until softened. Add the Swiss chard and garlic, then sauté until the chard leaves are wilted and the moisture has evaporated. Stir in the vinegar and cook for about 3 minutes, until the liquid has been absorbed. Stir in the pine nuts and then remove the pan from the heat. Season to taste.

Spoon into bowls and serve warm.

Shoestring sweet potato fries

{ *SERVES* 2 }

Something I've noticed on my journey through motherhood is the strange phenomenon of children accepting or rejecting food based on shape alone. It's amazing to see a young child reject a zucchini in standard form, but gleefully accept it once it's been spiralised into noodles. These shoestring sweet potato fries are another example of how form correlates directly with enjoyment. Kiddies and adults will adore their fine crunchy sweetness.

1 large sweet potato, peeled
2 tablespoons olive oil
sea salt, to taste

Preheat the oven to 200°C (400°F).

Slice the top off the sweet potato to make a flat surface (which makes spiralising easier). Spiralise the sweet potato according to the manufacturer's instructions. Arrange on a baking tray, toss with the olive oil and salt, and ensure you spread the noodles in a single layer.

Bake for 25 minutes, tossing halfway through cooking, or until the fries are tender and starting to crisp up and char at the edges.

Oven-baked broccoli and cauliflower steaks

{ *SERVES* 4 }

2 tablespoons extra virgin
olive oil

3 garlic cloves

2 tablespoons lemon juice

1 teaspoon cumin seeds

1 teaspoon ground coriander

1 teaspoon garam masala

½ teaspoon ground turmeric

2 tablespoons nutritional yeast
flakes

sea salt and freshly ground
black pepper, to taste

1 small head cauliflower, cut
into 4 thick slices

1 head broccoli, cut into 4 thick
slices

Sheep's Yoghurt Dip with
Pomegranate (page 259),
to serve

small handful coriander
(cilantro) leaves, to serve

Preheat the oven to 200°C (400°F) and line
a baking tray with baking paper.

In a small bowl, combine the olive oil, garlic,
lemon juice, cumin seeds, ground coriander,
garam masala, turmeric, yeast flakes, salt
and pepper.

Lay the cauliflower and broccoli slices on the
prepared baking tray, and brush with the spice
mixture, turning over to coat both sides. Bake
for 20–30 minutes, until tender. Set aside
to cool.

Transfer the 'steaks' to a plate, top with sheep's
yoghurt dip with pomegranate and garnish with
the coriander leaves to serve.

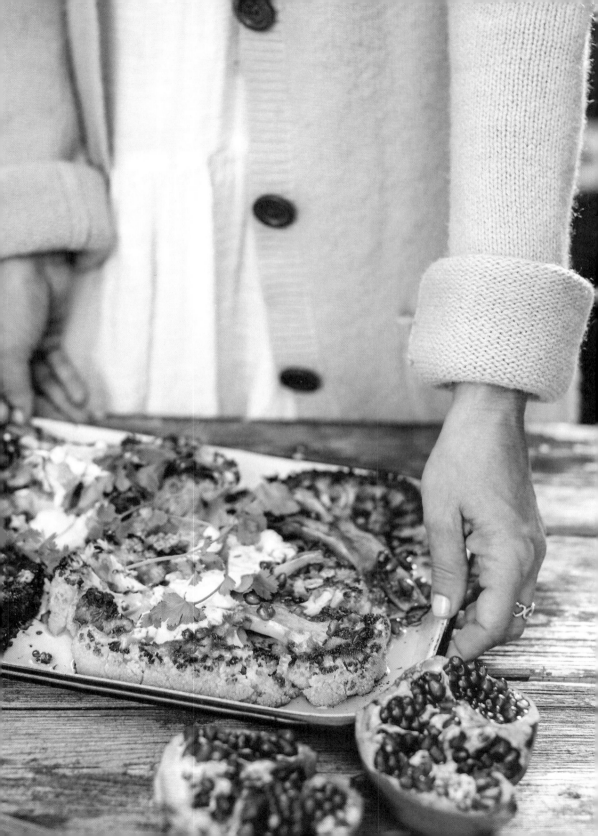

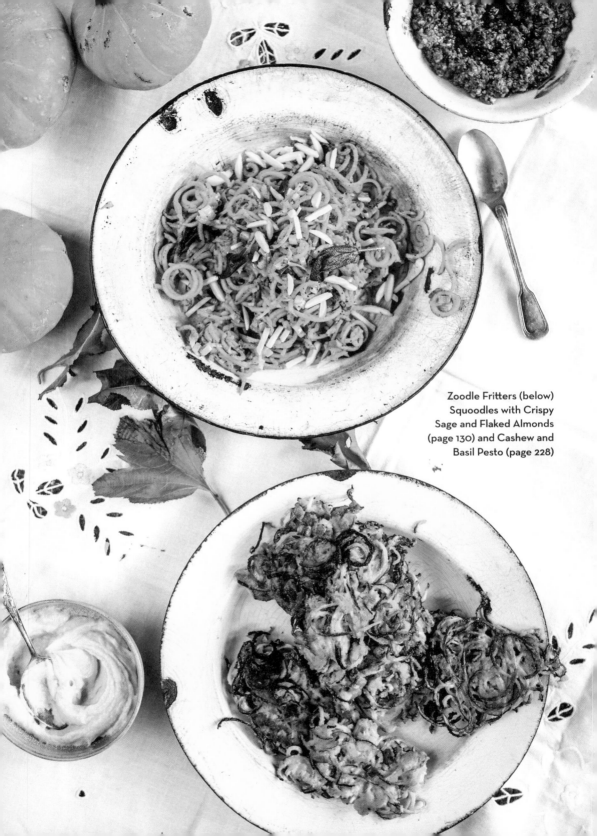

Zoodle Fritters (below)
Squoodles with Crispy
Sage and Flaked Almonds
(page 130) and Cashew and
Basil Pesto (page 228)

Zoodle fritters

{ *MAKES 24 SMALL OR 12 LARGE* }

540 g (1 lb 3 oz/4 cups)
  spiralised zucchini (courgette)

sea salt, as needed

100 g (3½ oz/1 cup) almond
  meal

2 large eggs, lightly beaten

1 garlic clove, crushed

2 spring onions (scallions),
  sliced

freshly ground black pepper,
  to taste

coconut oil, for frying

Lemony Goat's Cheese Dip
  (page 256), to serve (optional)

Put the spiralised zucchini in a colander, sprinkle with salt, leave to drain for about 20 minutes, then squeeze out any excess moisture with your hands.

Transfer the zucchini to a bowl, add the almond meal, eggs, garlic, spring onions, salt and pepper, and stir until well combined.

Line a plate with paper towel. Liberally coat the bottom of a large frying pan with coconut oil and heat over medium–high heat. Scoop 60 g (2¼ oz/¼ cup) mounds of the zucchini mixture into the pan, pressing them lightly into rounds at least 5 cm (2 inches) apart. Cook for 4 minutes on each side, or until golden brown and cooked through. Transfer to the paper-lined plate and repeat with the remaining zucchini mixture.

Serve the fritters as a side or with lemony goat's cheese dip.

Squoodles with crispy sage and flaked almonds

{ *SERVES* 2-3 }

1 small butternut pumpkin
   (squash) or pumpkin (winter
   squash), halved, peeled and
   seeds removed
50 ml (1¾ fl oz) coconut oil
½ teaspoon freshly grated
   nutmeg
½ teaspoon ground cinnamon
sea salt and freshly ground
   black pepper, to taste
12 sage leaves
olive oil, for drizzling
1 leek, pale part only, sliced
3 garlic cloves, sliced
juice of 1 lemon
35 g (1¼ oz/¼ cup) slivered
   almonds
20 g (¾ oz/¼ cup) nutritional
   yeast flakes
Cashew and Basil Pesto
   (page 228), to serve

Preheat the oven to 200°C (400°F) and line two baking trays with baking paper.

Spiralise the pumpkin using the large noodle attachment on your spiraliser or shave thinly with a vegetable peeler to make squoodles.

Transfer to one of the prepared baking trays, massage with half the coconut oil, then sprinkle over the spices, salt and pepper. Bake for about 10 minutes, until soft.

Meanwhile, lay the sage leaves on the second baking tray, drizzle with olive oil and roast for 5 minutes, or until crispy.

Heat the remaining coconut oil in a frying pan over medium heat, and sauté the leek and garlic until soft and translucent. Stir through the squoodles then add the lemon juice and almonds, tossing well to coat. Divide between serving bowls, top with the roasted sage leaves and sprinkle over the nutritional yeast flakes.

Serve with cashew and basil pesto on the side.

Chargrilled vegie stack with avocado dressing

{ SERVES 6 }

125 ml (4 fl oz/½ cup) olive oil

60 ml (2 fl oz/¼ cup) apple cider vinegar

3 garlic cloves, chopped

2 tablespoons lemon juice

1 tablespoon mixed dried herbs (e.g. thyme, basil, parsley)

6 large portobello mushrooms, stems removed

1 eggplant (aubergine), trimmed and cut into 6 slices

2 red capsicums (peppers), seeded and cut into 3 slices

2 yellow capsicums (peppers), seeded and cut into 3 slices

1 large zucchini (courgette), halved lengthways and cut into thirds to make 6 pieces

2 large tomatoes, cut into 6 slices

1 butternut pumpkin (squash), halved crossways, peeled, seeds removed, cut lengthways into 6 slices

1 large red onion, cut into 6 slices

sea salt and freshly ground black pepper, to taste

Avocado dressing

1 avocado, peeled

1 heaped teaspoon ground cumin

juice of 1 large lime

1 teaspoon lime zest

generous pinch of sea salt

2 tablespoons filtered water

1 tablespoon cold-pressed extra virgin olive oil

To make the avocado dressing, blend all the ingredients except the olive oil in a food processor until smooth. With the motor still running, add the olive oil very slowly in a thin stream until the mixture has the desired creaminess. The dressing will keep for 3–4 days in an airtight container in the fridge.

Heat the grill (broiler) to medium.

In a glass jar, combine the olive oil, vinegar, garlic, lemon juice and dried herbs, then seal tightly and shake until well combined.

In a large bowl, combine the mushrooms, eggplant, capsicum, zucchini, tomato, pumpkin and onion. Pour in the olive oil and dried herb mixture, and stir gently to coat. Season with salt and pepper.

Lay the vegies on the oven grill tray and grill for 20–25 minutes, until cooked, turning once and checking frequently to remove faster-cooking vegetables.

To serve, layer the vegetables in a stack on each plate, starting with a mushroom, followed by a spoonful of avocado dressing; then eggplant, red and yellow capsicum and zucchini, and another spoonful of avocado dressing. Finish with tomato, pumpkin and onion and serve hot.

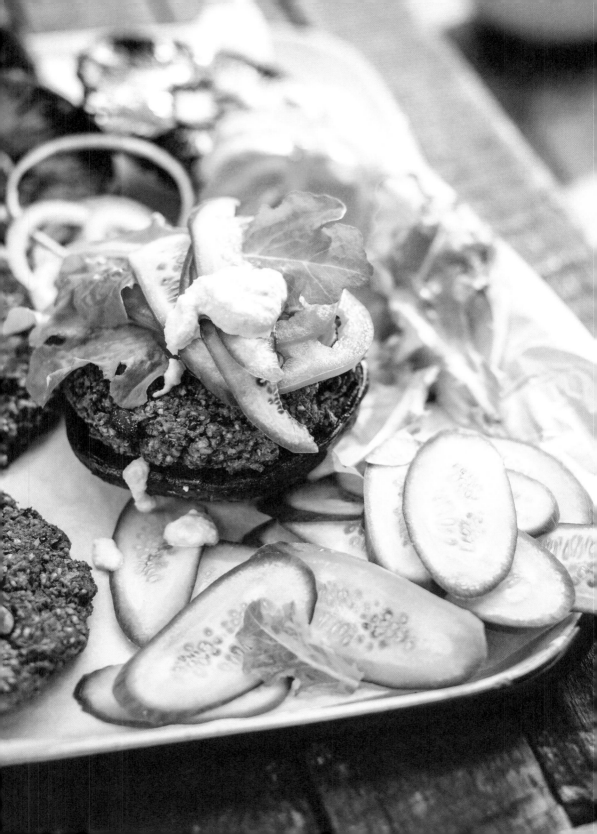

Portobello black bean burgers with lemon and garlic aioli

{ *SERVES* 4 }

These burgers are also delicious served with a pesto (pages 228–29) or wholegrain mustard.

60 ml (2 fl oz/¼ cup) coconut aminos or wheat-free tamari

1 teaspoon coconut sugar

1 tablespoon apple cider vinegar

4 large portobello mushrooms

20 g (¾ oz/½ tightly packed cup) rocket (arugula), washed and dried

4 thin slices red onion

2 tomatoes, sliced

½ cucumber, sliced

Black bean patties

75 g (2¾ oz/½ cup) sunflower seeds

75 g (2¾ oz/½ cup) pepitas (pumpkin seeds)

1 carrot, grated

400 g (14 oz) tinned black beans, rinsed and drained

1 brown onion, chopped

1 teaspoon ground cinnamon

1 teaspoon ground cumin

1 teaspoon ground coriander

½ teaspoon cayenne pepper

½ chilli, chopped

2 tablespoons cold-pressed extra virgin olive oil

sea salt and freshly ground black pepper, to taste

Lemon and garlic aioli (see tip, page 134)

2 egg yolks

4 large garlic cloves, crushed

1 tablespoon lemon juice, plus extra as needed

1 tablespoon filtered water

310 ml (10¾ fl oz/1¼ cups) light olive oil

sea salt, as needed

Continued page 134

If you prefer not to eat eggs, try this version of the aioli.

Egg-free lemon and garlic aioli

80 g (2³/₄ oz/¹/₂ cup) raw cashews, soaked in filtered water for 2 hours, drained

2 garlic cloves
pinch of sea salt
juice of 1 lemon
1 tablespoon filtered water

Blend all the ingredients in a food processor until creamy. This keeps for 4–5 days in an airtight container in the fridge.

To make the aioli, beat the egg yolks and garlic in a small bowl with a wooden spoon. Add the lemon juice and water, and keep beating. Slowly drizzle in the olive oil, beating continuously, until the mixture has the desired consistency. Add more lemon juice and sea salt to taste if needed. (Alternatively, prepare in a food processor.) The aioli will keep in a sterilised, tightly sealed jar in the fridge for up to 7 days.

Preheat the oven to 200°C (400°F) and lightly grease a baking tray.

To make the patties, pulse the sunflower seeds and pepitas in a food processor until coarsely chopped. Add the carrot and pulse for 10 seconds. Add three-quarters of the black beans, the onion, spices, chilli, olive oil, salt and pepper, then pulse again for 10 seconds. Stir the remaining beans into the mixture. Using your hands, shape portions of the mixture into four small patties and place them on the prepared baking tray. Bake for 20 minutes.

Meanwhile, make a marinade for the mushrooms by mixing the coconut aminos, coconut sugar and vinegar in a small bowl until the sugar has dissolved. Put the mushrooms in a large frying pan, generously spoon over the marinade, then place over medium heat until cooked through.

To assemble the burgers, place one mushroom on each plate, lay a black bean patty on top, then add the rocket, slices of onion, tomato and cucumber, and top with the aioli.

Asparagus with lemon-scented tahini dressing

{ *SERVES* 2 }

350 g (12 oz/2 bunches) asparagus, woody ends trimmed

1 tablespoon ghee, melted

a few tarragon sprigs, torn

freshly ground black pepper, to serve

Tahini dressing

65 g (2¼ oz/¼ cup) tahini

2 tablespoons lemon juice

1 teaspoon grated lemon zest

2 tablespoons wheat-free tamari

60 ml (2 fl oz/¼ cup) filtered water

Preheat the oven to 200°C (400°F).

To make the dressing, combine all the ingredients in a food processor and blend until smooth. Transfer to a glass jar and refrigerate for 30 minutes for the flavours to develop. Leftovers will keep for 4–5 days in an airtight container in the fridge.

Lay the asparagus in a roasting tin, toss with the ghee and roast for 5 minutes or until the asparagus just begins to brown and is al dente.

Drizzle the dressing over the roasted asparagus and toss gently to coat. Top with the tarragon, season with pepper and serve.

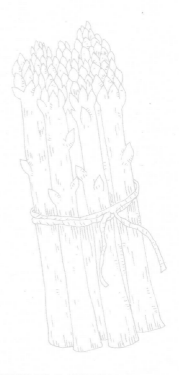

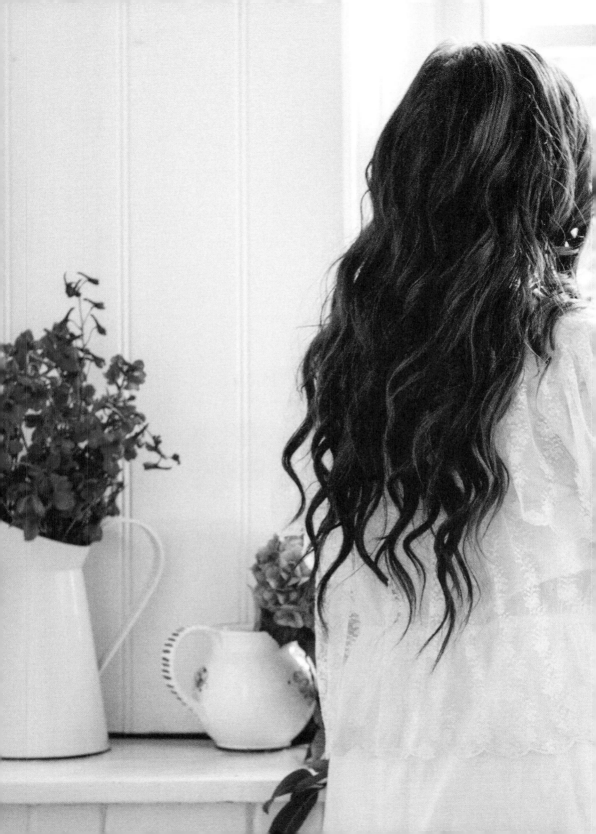

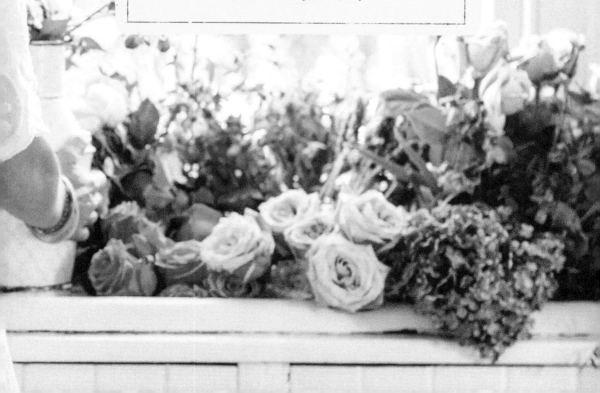

PART TWO

love

{ *PAGES 137—265* }

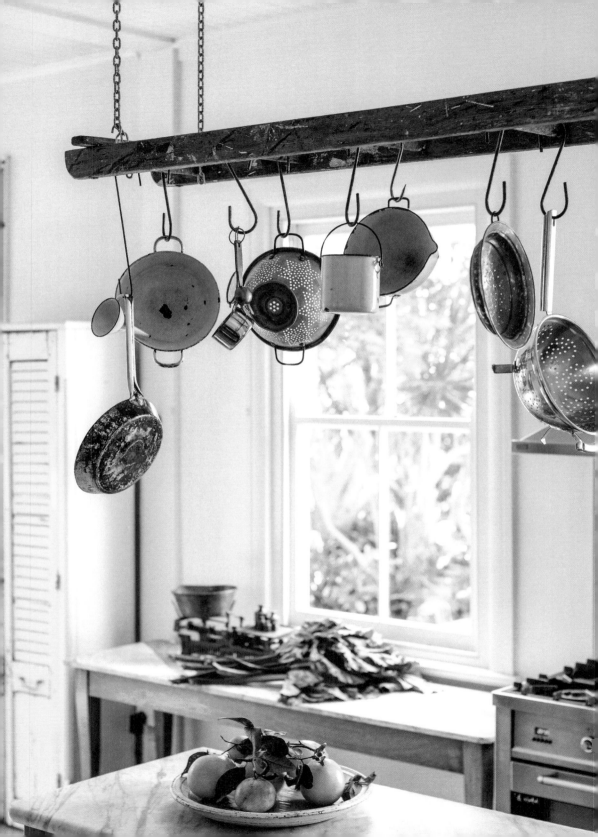

The heart of the home

At this point in history, we seem busier than ever. We outsource everything, including our food preparation. The definition of 'cooking' for the modern man or woman appears to include taking out a packet of pre-made ravioli and pre-made pasta sauce, heating them up and covering them with pre-grated cheese. This is a far cry from the home preparation of stocks, breads and other foods that our great-grandparents would have been involved in daily.

Previous generations were raised knowing where their food came from. They probably visited or lived on the farms where their fruit and vegetables grew, maybe even picked them from their own backyard, preserving the excess bounty as jams and pickles to be eaten in the months that followed. Not yet dictated to by a global market, they would have eaten seasonally, knowing that winter is a time for grounding root vegetable stews, and that spring brings the sweetest green peas and juicy lamb chops. Sadly for 21st-century generations, we've completely lost touch with our earth's seasonal wisdom and how it provides our body with exactly the nutrients and life forces it needs to flourish through the extremes.

Multinational food corporations and monstrous shopping centres are full of 'fresh' foods from all over the world, making it normal to purchase berries or citrus fruits year round. As a result, our bodies, hearts and souls have become confused, and because we're so busy being blindsided in the rat race of life – working, paying off debts and trying to get ahead – we cannot fully appreciate the beauty of a season's first fruits. Cooking has become less magical.

A KITCHEN WITH HEART

In a supercharged kitchen, true nourishment begins. There's so much potential, wherever you live, to create memories of love and hospitality that will linger in the imagination of your family and friends. The kitchen is where your food culture is established, where you decide on and store the kinds of ingredients you wish to share with your loved ones. You can either have a pantry full of pre-packaged foods, or a wondrous landscape of individual, fresh, organic, seasonal ingredients waiting to be combined into fulfilling, wholesome meals.

Many people find the kitchen a stressful place to be; some even despise cooking, preferring to fork out money for a convenient takeaway meal. The problem with this is you're not just paying for the food, you're paying for a business. The way many restaurant and takeaway businesses make their money is by minimising expenditure to increase their profit margin; in other words, they buy cheap, low-quality ingredients, make them taste good by coating them in additive-laden sauces and seasonings, then sell each dish at a price that allows their staff, rent and bills to be paid, with some extra on top for the business owners. I'd much rather put my money towards quality, ethically produced ingredients sourced from local producers and farmers' markets, add a little kitchen work and enjoy a meal that's better on my wallet, better for the planet, and better for my body and my family. You?

Food is at the heart of the home, and cooking is the vehicle to ensure a healthier and happier society. Michael Pollan famously addresses what he calls 'a curious paradox' around food in his book *Cooked*, where he observes that his fellow Americans seem to be devoting more time to *thinking* about food than ever before. An increasing interest in TV shows about food and cooking coincides with a collective disengagement from real food and the act of cooking in the home. With more meals prepared outside the home thanks to industrial food production, it seems the less Americans cook, the more interesting they find food and its preparation.

This is a slap in the face for all of us. If we're so transfixed by cooking that we spend hours gazing at, thinking about and observing it in the media, why as a society do we value our own kitchens so little? It's time we began to fall in love with the instinctive, natural, utterly human behaviour of cooking once again, and we can only fall in love with our kitchens when we rekindle our love for food. Food is central to the seven keystones of life, as discussed earlier, and this is where we need to begin our food safari – in the heart of the home.

I've gathered together a few of my favourite traditional recipes with a cultural twist, which I've collected on my travels to the United Kingdom, India, Asia, Europe and beyond. Whatever your food culture, be inspired to take a journey in your kitchen with these tasty meals and drinks.

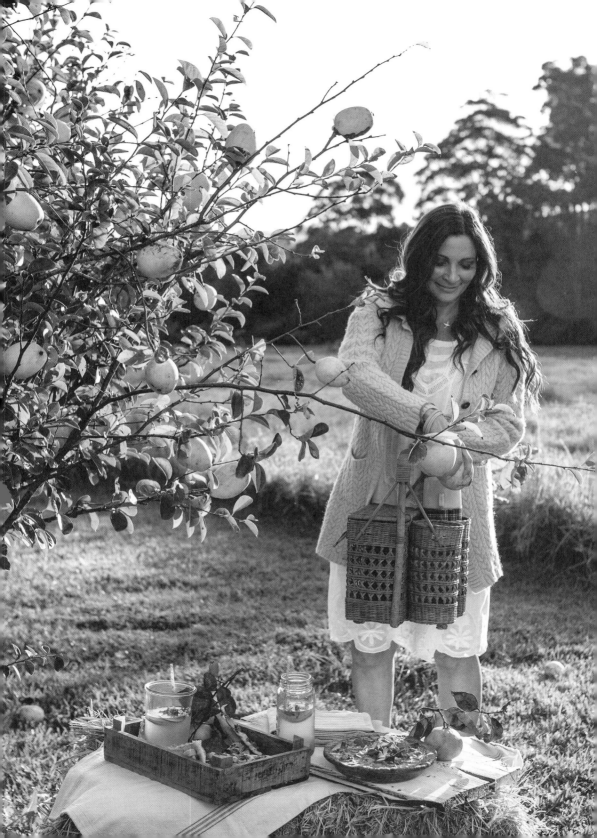

Mulled apple and berry cider

{ SERVES 2 }

500 ml (17 fl oz/2 cups) apple juice

220 g (7³/₄ oz/1 cup) mixed berries

6 cloves

2 cardamom pods, crushed

1 tablespoon rice malt syrup

2 cinnamon sticks

good pinch of freshly grated nutmeg, to serve

Pour the apple juice into a small saucepan. Add the remaining ingredients except the nutmeg, and warm gently over low heat, stirring frequently. Serve sprinkled with nutmeg (see note).

Note: The cider can be strained before serving if you prefer.

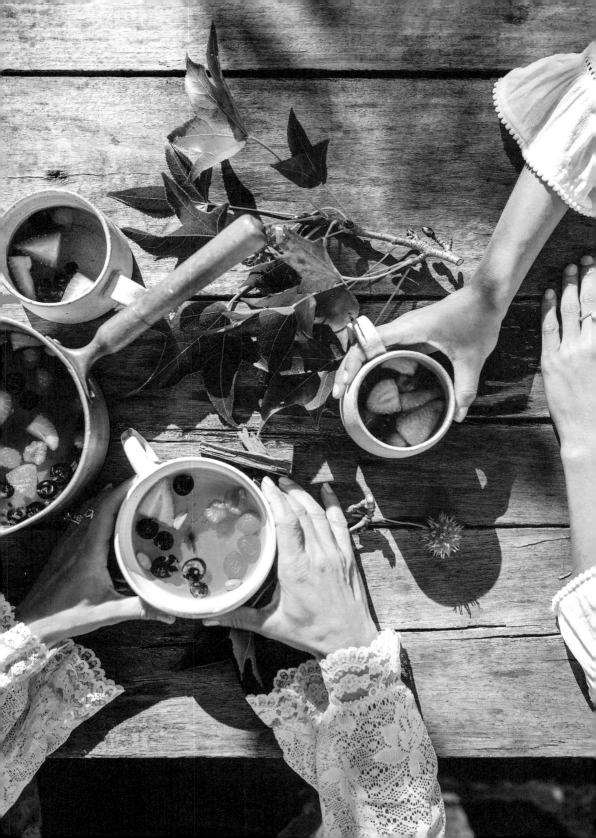

Indonesian-inspired banana omelette for two

{ SERVES 2 }

This recipe reminds me of the breakfast street food I enjoyed every morning when I was teaching English across Indonesia. You can make a savoury version too, with shallots, garlic, chilli and toasted shredded coconut. The sweet version also tastes sensational with in-season mango, chopped mint and toasted coconut.

2 large eggs

$\frac{1}{4}$ teaspoon ground cinnamon

$\frac{1}{4}$ teaspoon freshly grated nutmeg

1 tablespoon chia seeds

1 teaspoon alcohol-free vanilla extract

pinch of sea salt

2 ripe bananas, mashed

1 tablespoon coconut oil

110 g (3^3/$_4$ oz/^{1}/$_2$ cup) fresh mixed berries

2 tablespoons pistachio nut kernels

rice malt syrup, for drizzling

handful mint leaves

toasted shredded coconut, to serve (optional)

In a small bowl, beat the eggs, then mix in the cinnamon, nutmeg, chia seeds, vanilla and salt. Stir in the mashed banana.

Heat the coconut oil in a small frying pan over medium heat. Pour the egg mixture into the frying pan and cook until set on the bottom. Scatter over the berries and pistachios, and continue cooking until firm on top.

Carefully remove from the pan, drizzle over the rice malt syrup, top with the mint leaves and the shredded coconut, if using, and serve immediately.

Chicken galangal

{ *SERVES* 3-4 }

750 ml (26 fl oz/3 cups) chicken
  stock

800 ml (28 fl oz) coconut milk

3 garlic cloves, peeled

2 large lemongrass stems,
  trimmed, cut into 5 cm
  (2 inch) lengths and bruised

6 thin slices fresh galangal or
  fresh ginger

8 kaffir lime leaves, torn

1 small red chilli, seeded and
  thinly sliced

juice of 2 limes

60 ml (2 fl oz/¼ cup) wheat-
  free tamari

750 g (1 lb 10 oz) boneless,
  skinless chicken breasts, cut
  into thin strips

90 g (3¼ oz/1 cup) thinly sliced
  button mushrooms

small handful basil leaves,
  thinly sliced

sea salt, to taste (optional)

coriander (cilantro), to serve

In a large saucepan over medium heat,
warm the chicken stock, coconut milk, garlic,
lemongrass, galangal, lime leaves, chilli, lime
juice and tamari, and bring to the boil. Reduce
the heat to low and simmer, covered, for about
7 minutes.

Strain through a sieve into another saucepan
and discard all the solids. Add the chicken
breast and simmer for 5 minutes. Add
the mushrooms and simmer for a further
5 minutes. Add the basil and season with salt,
if needed.

Ladle into bowls and serve immediately,
garnished with coriander leaves.

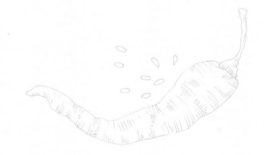

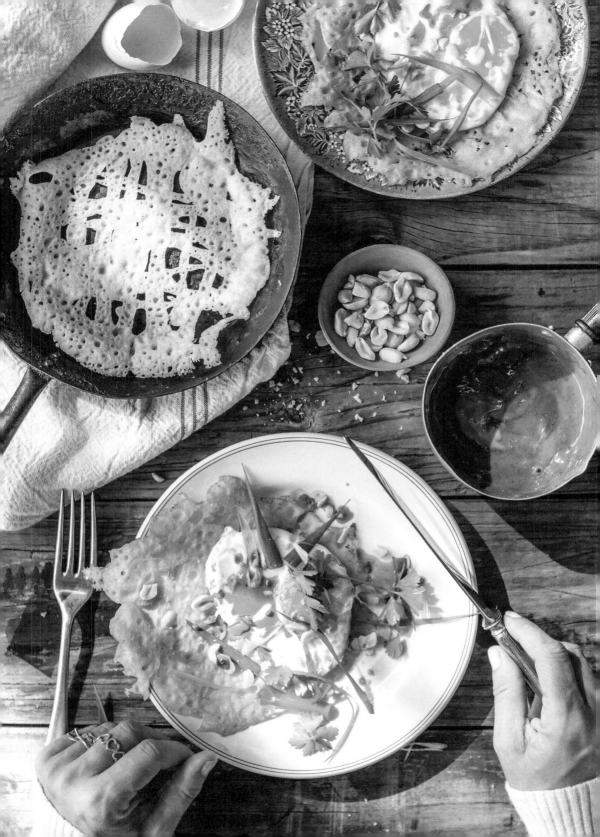

Egg hoppers

{ *SERVES 2* }

These cute, crepey edible 'bowls' are a popular way to serve street food in Sri Lanka, housing a variety of fillings from a fried egg to baked tomatoes topped with herbs or simply peanut sauce, coconut or sambal. My version doesn't include the typical yeast, so the lattice handiwork when pouring the batter into the pan helps to achieve the desired, if somewhat flatter shape.

1 egg, whisked

160 g (5¾ oz/1 cup) rice flour

375 ml (13 fl oz/1½ cups) coconut milk

pinch of sea salt

olive or coconut oil, for frying

Toppings

4 eggs

torn spring onions (scallions), roughly chopped peanuts, coriander (cilantro) leaves and lime wedges, to serve

Peanut sauce

70 g (2½ oz/¼ cup) natural peanut butter

2 tablespoons wheat-free tamari or coconut aminos

1 garlic clove, crushed

⅛ teaspoon grated fresh ginger

80 ml (2½ fl oz/⅓ cup) warm filtered water

To make the peanut sauce, combine all the ingredients in a small bowl and whisk until thoroughly mixed.

Beat the whisked egg, rice flour, coconut milk and salt together with a fork until smooth. Heat about 1 tablespoon olive oil in a small frying pan with rounded sides. Using a small spoon or squeeze bottle, drizzle about 60 ml (2 fl oz/ ¼ cup) of the batter over the base and sides of the pan in a thin layer, leaving holes in the mix (like the picture). Cook until bubbles form on the surface and the edges are golden, then remove carefully with a spatula and set aside. Repeat the process with the remaining batter.

Fry the eggs in a separate frying pan and place one on top of each hopper. Spoon over some peanut sauce, scatter over the spring onions, chopped peanuts and coriander, and serve with lime wedges.

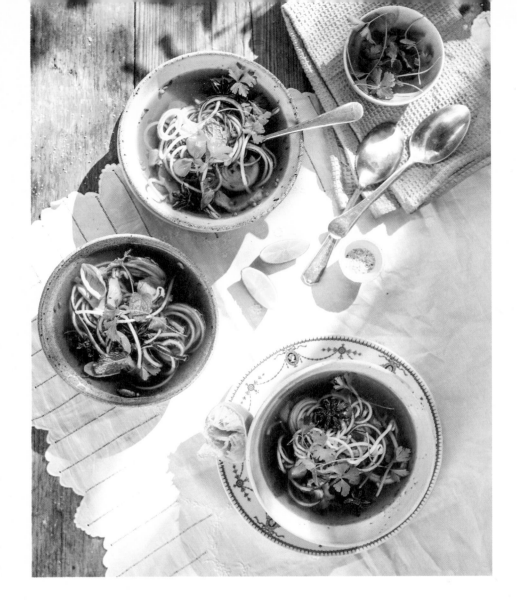

Beef pho bone broth

{ *SERVES* 4 }

Bone broth is all the rage at the moment, but you can enjoy the gelatinous benefits of this age-old tonic in a variety of delicious ways. This particular twist will whisk you away to the streets of northern Vietnam, where pho originated in the early 20th century. It was initially sold at dawn and dusk by roaming street vendors shouldering mobile kitchens. The garnish of lime and bean sprouts is a modern variation on this healing traditional broth.

1 tablespoon coconut oil

1 kg (2 lb 4 oz) beef bones (shin, knuckles, marrow and gelatinous cuts are good)

2 litres (68 fl oz/8 cups) filtered water, plus extra as needed

2 tablespoons apple cider vinegar

pinch of sea salt

6 star anise

2 cinnamon sticks

3 cardamom pods

2 teaspoons coriander seeds

2 teaspoons fennel seeds

3 cloves

1 brown onion, halved and sliced

1 × 7.5 cm (3 inch) piece fresh ginger, grated

1 tablespoon wheat-free tamari

500 g (1 lb 2 oz) beef (e.g. sirloin), thinly sliced

3 zucchini (courgettes), spiralised

To serve

handful bean sprouts, trimmed

handful mixed basil, mint and coriander (cilantro) leaves

2 limes, cut into wedges

Preheat the oven to 200°C (400°F).

Heat a large flameproof casserole dish over medium heat and melt the coconut oil. Add the bones and stir to coat. Cover and transfer the casserole dish to the oven for 30 minutes, or until the bones are browned.

Return the dish to the stovetop and add the water, vinegar and salt. Bring to the boil, then reduce the heat to as low as possible and simmer, covered, for 1½ hours, adding a little more water from time to time if necessary. Carefully remove the bones using tongs and discard. Allow the broth to cool, then skim any unwanted fat off the top, setting it aside.

Heat a heavy-based frying pan over medium heat and toast the spices for 2 minutes, or until fragrant. Move the spices to the side of the pan, add some of the reserved broth fat, then sauté the onion and ginger until the onion is translucent. Transfer to the casserole dish with the stock then add the tamari and beef. Return to a gentle boil over medium heat on the stovetop, then reduce the heat to low, add the zucchini noodles and simmer for 5 minutes, or until the noodles are al dente.

Ladle into bowls, top with the bean sprouts, garnish with the herbs and serve with the lime wedges.

SUPERCHARGED TIP

If you have a slow-cooker, it's perfect for this pho. If you prefer your noodles crunchier and your beef rare, you can put the noodles and beef into the bowls then pour over the hot broth.

Lamb mulligatawny

{ *SERVES* 4-6 }

2 tablespoons coconut oil

1 large brown onion, finely chopped

2 carrots, finely chopped

2 celery stalks, thinly sliced

1 × 2 cm (³/₄ inch) piece fresh ginger, grated

4 large garlic cloves, crushed

2 teaspoons ground turmeric

2 teaspoons ground ginger

¹/₂ teaspoon freshly ground black pepper

¹/₂ teaspoon paprika

1 teaspoon ground coriander

1 teaspoon ground cumin

¹/₂ teaspoon black mustard seeds

750 g (1 lb 10 oz) lamb, cut into 2 cm (³/₄ inch) dice

500 ml (17 fl oz/2 cups) stock or filtered water

1 bay leaf

1 teaspoon lemon zest

juice of 1 grated lemon

few thyme sprigs

2 teaspoons sea salt

Coconut 'Yoghurt' (page 195) and coriander (cilantro) or fresh curry leaves (optional), to serve

Heat the coconut oil in a large saucepan and sauté the onion, carrot, celery, ginger and garlic for 4-5 minutes, until the onion is translucent. Stir in the spices and cook for 2 minutes, or until fragrant. Add the lamb and cook until brown. Stir in the stock and bring to the boil, then add the bay leaf, reduce the heat to low and simmer gently, covered, for 1 hour 15 minutes.

Add the lemon zest and juice and the thyme, then simmer for an additional 10 minutes. Season to taste.

To serve, swirl in some coconut 'yoghurt' and garnish with coriander.

SUPERCHARGED TIP

You could bulk up the dish by adding some cooked buckwheat or quinoa.

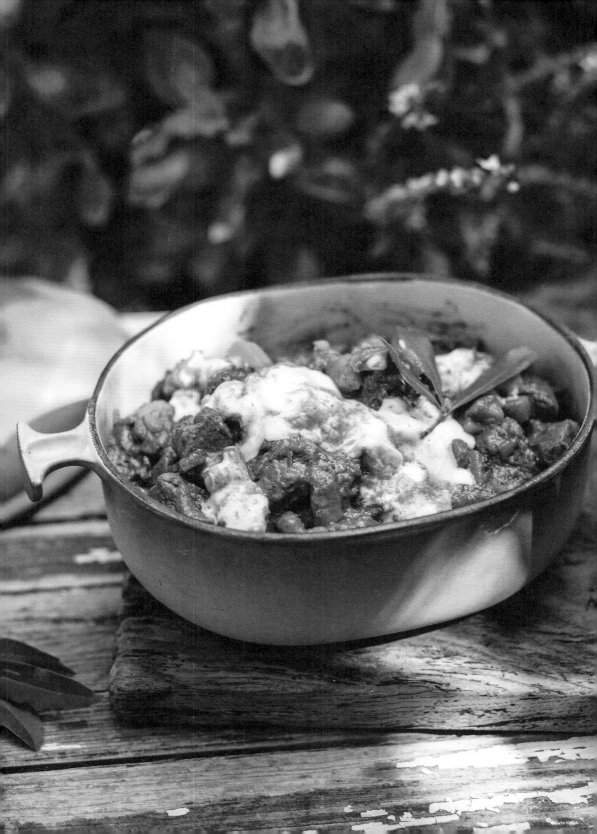

Caesar salad with nachos crackers

{ *SERVES* 4 }

dash of apple cider vinegar

4 eggs

16 nitrate-free prosciutto slices

1 large cos (romaine) lettuce,
washed, dried and torn

12 anchovy fillets

20 g (³/₄ oz/¹/₄ cup) nutritional
yeast flakes or 1 quantity
Cashew Cheese (page 288)

sea salt and freshly ground
black pepper, to taste

Nachos crackers

100 g (3¹/₂ oz/1 cup) almond meal

1 large egg

1 teaspoon ground turmeric

¹/₄ teaspoon ground cumin

¹/₄ teaspoon ground coriander

1 teaspoon grated orange zest

1 teaspoon sea salt

Caesar dressing

65 g (2¹/₄ oz/¹/₄ cup) almond
butter

2 small garlic cloves, finely
chopped

20 g (³/₄ oz/¹/₄ cup) nutritional
yeast flakes

60 ml (2 fl oz/¹/₄ cup) lemon
juice

60 g (2¹/₄ oz/¹/₄ cup) dijon mustard

60 ml (2 fl oz/¹/₄ cup) filtered
water

2 tablespoons wheat-free tamari

2 tablespoons flaxseed oil

freshly ground black pepper,
to taste

Preheat the oven to 180°C (350°F).

To make the crackers, combine all the ingredients in a large bowl and mix with a wooden spoon to form a dough.

Lay a sheet of baking paper on a clean work surface, place the dough on top, then cover with a second sheet of baking paper. Roll the dough out to 2 mm (¹/₁₆ inch) thick. Remove the top piece of baking paper and transfer the dough on the bottom piece of baking paper to a baking tray. Using a sharp knife, deeply score the dough into 3 cm (1¹/₄ inch) squares.

Bake for 12 minutes. Allow to cool before breaking into crackers.

For the dressing, mix all the ingredients in a small bowl and set aside.

Bring a medium saucepan of water to the boil, add the vinegar and poach the eggs to your liking. Meanwhile, crisp up the prosciutto in a large heavy-based frying pan.

Toss the lettuce with the dressing in a large bowl. Add the eggs, prosciutto and anchovies, sprinkle over the yeast flakes or cashew cheese, top with the nachos crackers and season with salt and pepper.

Niçoise salad with baked herb-crusted salmon

{ *SERVES* 4 }

200 g (7 oz) green beans

4 eggs, soft-boiled

4 vine-ripened tomatoes

8 anchovy fillets

135 g (4³⁄₄ oz/3 cups) baby English spinach leaves

175 g (6 oz) small black olives

Herb-crusted salmon

2 spring onions (scallions)

2 tablespoons chopped flat-leaf (Italian) parsley

2 tablespoons chopped basil

2 teaspoons chopped oregano

2 teaspoons chopped thyme

2 large garlic cloves, crushed

1 teaspoon sea salt

freshly ground black pepper, to taste

2 tablespoons extra virgin olive oil, plus extra as needed

4 × 150 g (5¹⁄₂ oz) salmon fillets, skin and bones removed

1 tablespoon dijon mustard

Mustard vinaigrette

60 ml (2 fl oz/¹⁄₄ cup) apple cider vinegar

1 tablespoon finely chopped red onion

1 tablespoon dijon mustard

1 tablespoon rice malt syrup or ¹⁄₂ teaspoon stevia powder

¹⁄₂ teaspoon sea salt

freshly ground black pepper, to taste

125 ml (4 fl oz/¹⁄₂ cup) extra virgin olive oil

1 tablespoon chopped basil

To make the vinaigrette whiz all the ingredients except the oil and basil in a blender or food processor. With the machine running, gradually drizzle in the olive oil to form an emulsion.

Add the basil and pulse to combine.

Preheat the oven to 230°C (450°F) and line a baking tray with baking paper.

To make the baked salmon, finely chop the spring onions, including the light green parts, mix with the herbs, garlic, salt and pepper in a small bowl, and stir in the oil. If the mixture is too dry, add a little more oil. Lay the salmon on the prepared baking tray. Using a small spatula or the back of a spoon, spread 1 teaspoon of the mustard over each fillet, then spoon the herb mixture on top and press down evenly with the back of a spoon. Bake the salmon for 8–10 minutes, until cooked to your liking.

Top and tail the beans and cut into 4–5 cm (1¹⁄₂–2 inch) lengths and either steam or blanch until crispy-tender. Rinse under cold running water to arrest the cooking process and set aside to cool. Peel the eggs and cut into quarters. Cut the tomatoes into wedges and slice the anchovies lengthways.

Arrange the spinach leaves on a serving platter and scatter around the beans, tomatoes, anchovies and olives. Tuck the eggs in and around the salad and then top with the salmon fillets. Drizzle the vinaigrette all over and serve immediately.

Okra tempura

{ *SERVES* 4 }

1 large egg yolk

250 ml (9 fl oz/1 cup) ice-cold soda water (club soda)

260 g (9¼ oz/2 cups) tapioca flour

½ teaspoon sea salt

extra virgin coconut oil, for frying

160 g (5¾ oz/2 cups) okra, caps removed, halved lengthways

Asian dipping sauce

2 tablespoons rice malt syrup

2 tablespoons wheat-free tamari

2 tablespoons lime juice

1 teaspoon chilli flakes

To make the dipping sauce, combine all the ingredients in a small saucepan and bring to the boil over medium–high heat. Cook, stirring constantly, for about 5 minutes, until the sauce is reduced by half. Pour into a small bowl and set aside.

Whisk the egg yolk and soda water in a medium bowl, then slowly whisk in the tapioca flour and salt to make a thin batter.

Heat some coconut oil (to about 4 cm/ 1½ inches deep) in a medium heavy-based saucepan over medium–high heat. Once the oil is hot enough for a small piece of okra to sizzle and float, working in batches, dip the okra in the batter to coat well, then fry until crisp all over. Lay on paper towel to drain off any excess oil while you cook the next batch.

Serve with the dipping sauce.

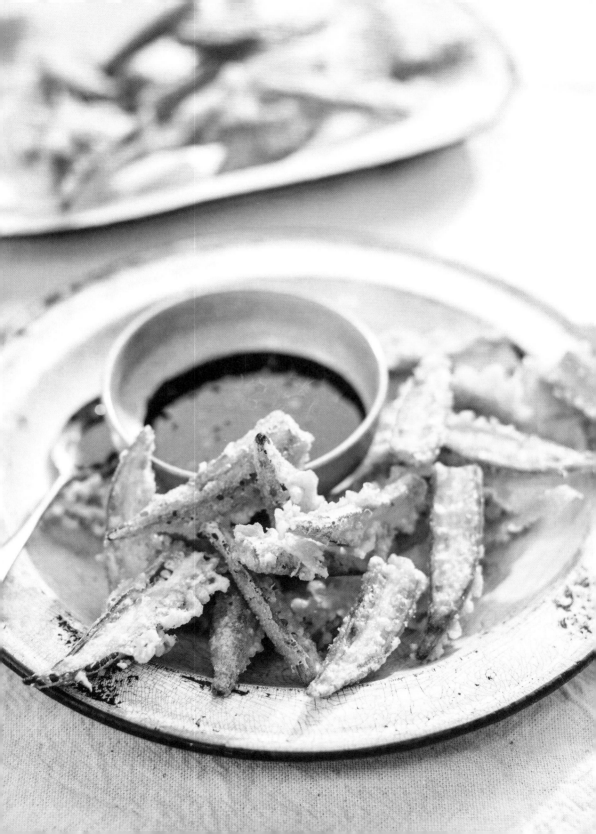

Rogan josh

{ *SERVES* 4–6 }

I have a serious thing going on with curries. My love affair with spices and their power to create such unique mixes of flavours inspires me. My spice rack is the most important section of my kitchen. You can't go past a classic Indian rogan josh to begin your home-made curry adventure. This is a great freezer meal to cook in batches and store in portions for midweek dinners.

750 g (1 lb 10 oz) lamb shoulder, cut into 2.5 cm (1 inch) dice

salt and freshly ground black pepper, to taste

1 tablespoon coconut oil

2 brown onions, diced

2 garlic cloves, chopped

250 ml (9 fl oz/1 cup) coconut milk

250 ml (9 fl oz/1 cup) coconut water

Cauliflower Rice (page 166), to serve

coconut flakes, to serve

handful coriander (cilantro) leaves, chopped

Spice blend

2 cloves

2 tablespoons sweet paprika

1 tablespoon ground cumin

1 tablespoon ground coriander

2 teaspoons chilli powder

2 teaspoons ground cinnamon

1 teaspoon ground cardamom

1 teaspoon grated fresh ginger

1 teaspoon cayenne pepper

1 teaspoon sea salt

To make the spice blend, mix all the spices in a small bowl (or mix into a paste in a mini-blender with a little coconut milk).

In a medium bowl, combine the lamb with salt and pepper, tossing with your hands.

Heat the coconut oil in a large saucepan or flameproof casserole dish over medium–high heat. Working in batches, sear the lamb on all sides until it is brown and the outside has a slight crust. Remove and set aside.

Add the onion and garlic to the same pan, and cook for 3–4 minutes, stirring, until the onion is translucent. Add the spice blend and stir for about 1 minute, until fragrant. Increase the heat to high, pour in the coconut milk and coconut water, return the lamb to the pan, mix well and bring to the boil. Reduce the heat to low and simmer, covered, for 1 hour, or until the lamb is fork-tender, then remove the lid and cook for another 30 minutes to thicken the sauce.

Serve with cauliflower rice and top with coconut flakes and coriander.

Mexican lamb shoulder with cumin, oregano and pomegranate glaze

{ *SERVES* 6–8 }

2 kg (4 lb 8 oz) bone-in lamb shoulder joint

2 brown onions, cut into wedges

1 garlic bulb

1 litre (35 fl oz/4 cups) pomegranate juice

juice of 1 lemon

60 ml (2 fl oz/¼ cup) apple cider vinegar

2 tablespoons rice malt syrup, plus extra as needed

1 pomegranate

250 g (9 oz) full-fat plain yoghurt

small handful mint leaves, chopped

Cashew and Basil Pesto (page 228; optional) and steamed green vegetables, to serve

Garlic marinade

4 garlic cloves, chopped

2 teaspoons ground cinnamon

2 teaspoons ground cumin

1 tablespoon dried oregano

grated zest and juice of 1 lemon

1 teaspoon sea salt

1 teaspoon freshly ground black pepper

Blend all of the marinade ingredients in a food processor until smooth.

Lay the lamb in a large baking dish, spoon the garlic marinade over the top and massage in using your hands. Cover and refrigerate for 2–24 hours to marinate.

Preheat the oven to 160°C (315°F).

Lay the lamb in a roasting tin, surround with the onion and garlic bulb, then pour over the pomegranate juice, lemon juice and vinegar. Cover the tin with foil, then roast for about 4 hours, basting every hour.

When ready, remove from the oven, carefully lift out the lamb, pour the juices into a saucepan, then return the lamb to the roasting tin, cover again with the foil and return to the oven.

Place the saucepan over medium heat. Add the rice malt syrup and boil until the mixture thickens, adding more rice malt syrup if necessary. This should take about 25 minutes. Once it is ready, remove the lamb from the oven, take off the foil, pour over the sauce and return to the oven for 20 minutes, or until the lamb is crispy on top.

Remove the seeds from the pomegranate. In a small bowl mix the yoghurt, pomegranate seeds and mint.

Serve the lamb with the yoghurt dressing, cashew and basil pesto, if using, and a side of steamed green vegetables.

Chermoula prawn and shaved fennel salad

{ *SERVES* 4 }

16 large prawns (shrimp),
   peeled and deveined, heads
   and tails left intact

Chermoula

1 teaspoon cumin seeds

1 teaspoon coriander seeds

1 teaspoon sweet paprika

1 × 2.5 cm (1 inch) piece fresh
   ginger, chopped

3 garlic cloves, roughly
   chopped

1 small red chilli, seeded and
   roughly chopped

handful parsley leaves

handful coriander (cilantro)
   leaves

1 tablespoon lemon juice

100 ml (3½ fl oz) olive oil

½ teaspoon sea salt

½ teaspoon freshly ground
   black pepper

Shaved fennel salad

2 tablespoons extra virgin olive
   oil

2 tablespoons lemon juice

¾ teaspoon sea salt

¼ teaspoon freshly black
   ground pepper

1 zucchini (courgette) or
   cucumber, thinly sliced
   lengthways using a vegetable
   peeler, mandoline or knife

1 large fennel bulb, fronds
   reserved and chopped, bulb
   shaved using a vegetable
   peeler, mandoline or knife

40 g (1½ oz) red onion, thinly
   sliced

To make the chermoula, process all the ingredients in a food processor until smooth.

Place the prawns in a bowl and add three-quarters of the chermoula, setting aside the rest in a jar in the fridge for later use. Mix until the prawns are well coated, then leave in the fridge to marinate for 1 hour.

Preheat a barbecue grill plate to high or heat a chargrill pan over medium–high heat and cook the prawns for 3–4 minutes on each side, until cooked through.

To make the salad, whisk the olive oil, lemon juice, salt and pepper in a large bowl. Add the zucchini, shaved fennel, half the fennel fronds and the onion, then stir gently to coat well.

Serve the prawns with the salad, and garnish with the remaining fennel fronds.

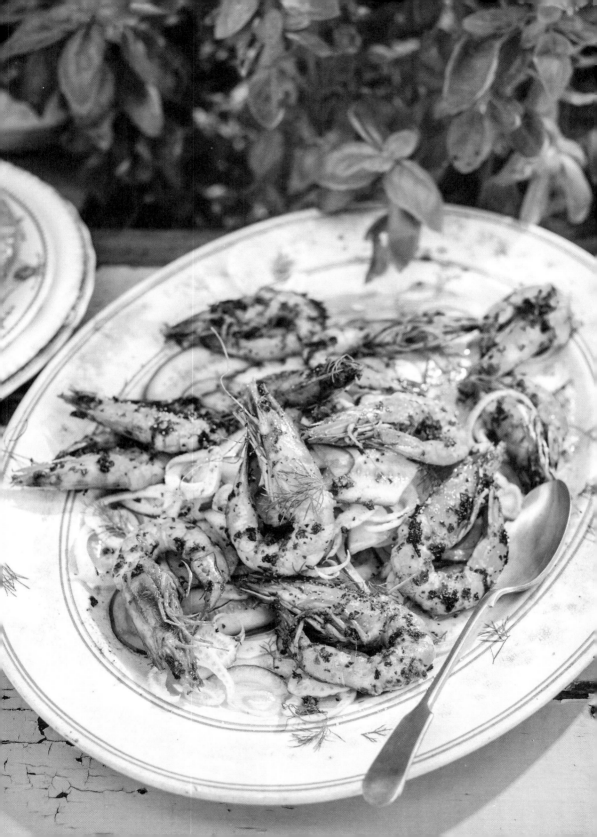

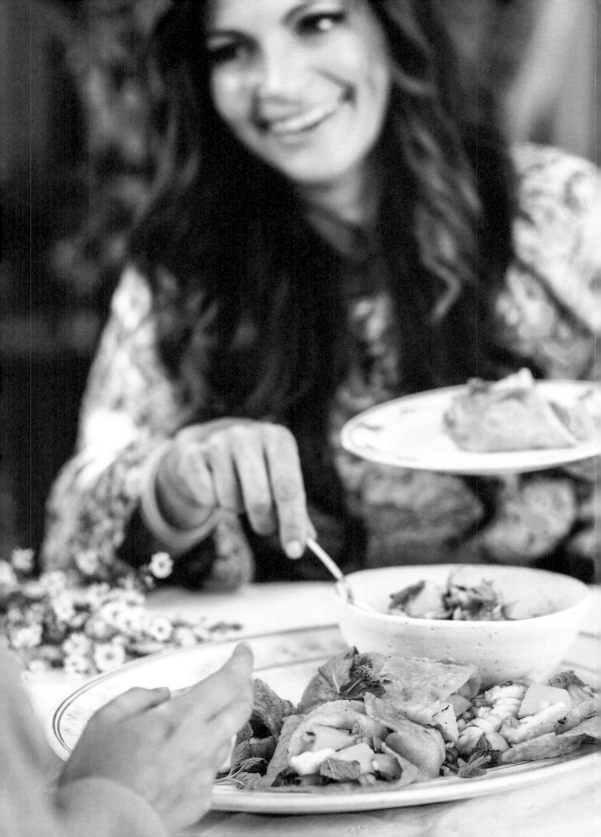

Fish tortillas

{ *MAKES* 4 }

4 firm white fish fillets

sea salt and freshly
   ground black pepper

juice of 1 lemon

1 avocado, peeled

1 tablespoon olive oil

100 g (3½ oz/2¾ tightly packed
   cups) rocket (arugula) or
   baby lettuce

2 ripe tomatoes, chopped

Dressing

1 red onion, finely diced

1 mango, peeled and diced

good handful coriander
   (cilantro) leaves, chopped
   (optional)

good handful mint leaves,
   chopped

2 tablespoons lime juice

1 tablespoon extra virgin olive
   oil

1 long red chilli, seeded and
   chopped (optional)

Tortillas

175 g (6 oz/1⅓ cups) tapioca
   flour

330 ml (11¼ fl oz/1⅓ cups)
   coconut milk

1 egg

pinch of sea salt

80 g (2¾ oz) butter

Season the fish with salt and pepper and splash half the lemon juice over the top. Set aside for 10 minutes.

Meanwhile, mash the avocado, adding the remaining lemon juice to taste to stop it turning brown.

To make the dressing, mix all the ingredients in a bowl and refrigerate for a little for the flavours to develop.

To make the tortillas, combine all the ingredients except the butter in a medium bowl, mixing well. Heat one-quarter of the butter in a medium frying pan over medium heat. Pour in 125 ml (4 fl oz/½ cup) of the mixture and swirl to cover the bottom of the pan. After 2–3 minutes, carefully turn over and brown the other side. Repeat with the remaining butter and tortilla mixture.

Heat the olive oil in a large frying pan and cook the fish for 3 minutes on each side, or until cooked through. Transfer to a plate and flake into large chunks.

To assemble, spread avocado on each tortilla, then add rocket and tomato, and top with fish pieces. Spoon the dressing over and then serve immediately.

Pork bibimbab

{ SERVES 3 }

1 large daikon (mooli), peeled and roughly chopped

2 tablespoons coconut oil, plus extra as needed

500 g (1 lb 2 oz) minced (ground) pork

60 ml (2 fl oz/$\frac{1}{4}$ cup) coconut aminos or wheat-free tamari, or to taste

3 garlic cloves, sliced

bunch spring onions (scallions), chopped

1 × 2.5 cm (1 inch) piece fresh ginger, grated

1 long red chilli, seeded and finely chopped

2 zucchini (courgettes), spiralised or cut into thin strips

2 teaspoons toasted sesame oil, plus extra to serve

120 g (4$\frac{1}{4}$ oz/2$\frac{2}{3}$ cups) baby English spinach leaves

3 eggs

1 cucumber, shaved thinly using a vegetable peeler

1 tablespoon sesame seeds, toasted

sea salt and freshly ground black pepper, to taste

In a food processor, chop the daikon into rice-sized pieces. Using your hands, squeeze out any excess moisture then set aside in a bowl.

Heat half the coconut oil in a wok or frying pan over medium heat, then add the pork and cook until it colours, using a wooden spoon to break up and stir the meat. Add the coconut aminos, garlic, spring onion (reserving a little for a garnish), ginger and chilli, and cook until the pork is cooked through and browned to your liking. Transfer to a bowl and cover.

Heat the remaining coconut oil in the same pan, then add the daikon, spreading it out evenly, and cook for 5–7 minutes, stirring frequently. Turn out into a bowl, then cook the zucchini for 8 minutes, adding more coconut oil if necessary. Transfer to a bowl and cover.

Heat the sesame oil in the same pan over medium heat, cook the spinach for a couple of minutes until wilted, then transfer to a bowl.

Add a little more coconut oil to the same pan, then fry the eggs until the whites are set and the yolks are still runny.

Divide the pork, daikon rice, spinach, cucumber and zucchini noodles between three bowls. Top each with a fried egg, then scatter over the reserved spring onions and the sesame seeds, season with salt and pepper, add a drop of extra sesame oil, and serve.

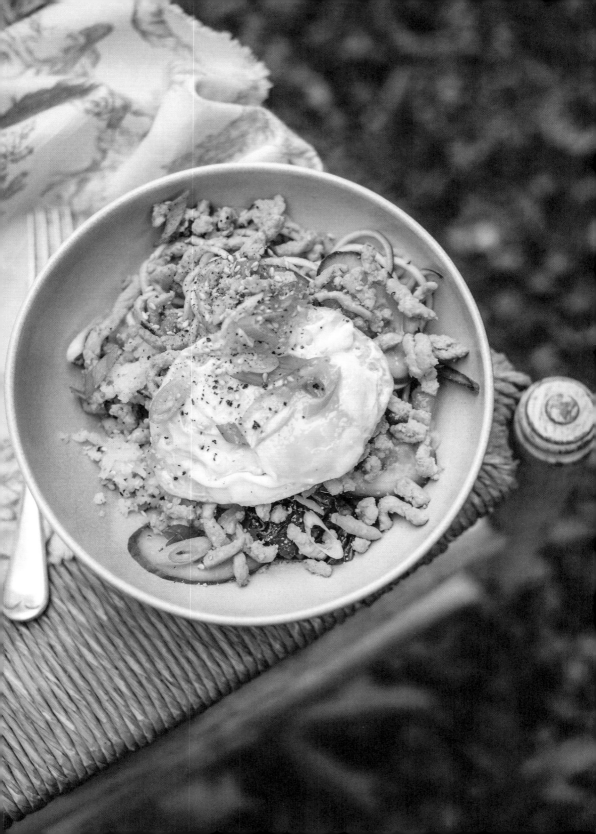

Prawn quinoa paella

{ *SERVES* 4 }

If you want a taste of traditional Spanish cuisine, it's hard to find a better pick than paella. This savoury dish, synonymous with Spanish culture and tradition, can highlight the flavours of fresh seafood from your local fishmonger. Typically served straight from the pan on a communal table, paella is a lovely dish for bringing people together.

1 tablespoon olive oil

1 brown onion, chopped

3 garlic cloves, crushed

1 long red chilli, seeded and finely chopped

1 red capsicum (pepper), seeded and chopped

300 g (10½ oz/1½ cups) quinoa, thoroughly rinsed and drained

pinch of saffron threads

1 teaspoon sweet paprika

1 teaspoon ground turmeric

½ teaspoon ground cumin

2 thyme sprigs, leaves picked

750 ml (26 fl oz/3 cups) vegetable or chicken stock

grated zest and juice of 1 lemon

155 g (5½ oz) fresh or frozen peas

4 large tomatoes, chopped

500 g (1 lb 2 oz) raw prawns (shrimp), peeled and deveined

sea salt and freshly ground black pepper, to taste

handful flat-leaf (Italian) parsley, roughly chopped

lemon wedges, to serve

Heat the olive oil in a deep heavy-based frying pan over medium heat and sauté the onion, garlic, chilli and capsicum for 5–6 minutes, until the onion is translucent. Add the quinoa and cook for 2 minutes, stirring. Add the spices, thyme and three-quarters of the vegetable stock. Bring to the boil, then reduce the heat to very low and simmer, covered, for 15 minutes, occasionally checking if the stock needs topping up.

Once the quinoa is cooked, add the lemon zest and juice, peas, tomatoes and prawns, and simmer until the prawns are cooked and all the liquid has been absorbed. Season with salt and pepper, stir through the parsley and serve with the lemon wedges.

Meatloaf laksa with rice noodles

{ *SERVES* 4 }

1 tablespoon coconut oil

1 brown onion, diced

1 × 1 cm (½ inch) piece fresh ginger, grated

1 tablespoon sugar-free laksa paste

375 ml (13 fl oz/1½ cups) coconut milk

750 ml (26 fl oz/3 cups) beef or vegetable stock or filtered water

handful coriander (cilantro) leaves, finely chopped, plus extra to serve

½ teaspoon curry powder

½ teaspoon chilli flakes, or to taste, plus extra to serve (optional)

sea salt and freshly ground black pepper, to taste

200 g (7 oz) rice noodles

60 g (2¼ oz/1 cup) broccoli florets

large handful snow peas (mangetout)

4 slices left-over Meatloaf (page 202)

Heat the coconut oil in a large saucepan or stockpot over medium–high heat and sauté the onion for 3–4 minutes, until translucent. Stir through the ginger and laksa paste, then add the coconut milk, stock, coriander, curry powder, chilli flakes, salt and pepper, and bring to the boil. Reduce the heat to medium–low and simmer for 5 minutes.

Add the rice noodles and cook for the time indicated on the packet. When the noodles are 2 minutes off being ready, add the broccoli and snow peas, then cook for 2 minutes, or until the greens are just cooked through without becoming too soft or losing their colour.

Cut each meatloaf slice into four squares and arrange in four deep serving plates or wide bowls. Using tongs, remove clumps of noodles from the laksa and arrange in a spiral on top of the meatloaf. Distribute the broccoli and snow peas evenly between the plates and then pour the laksa liquid over, distributing all the ingredients as equally as possible.

Garnish with extra coriander, and a little salt and pepper. Serve with extra chilli flakes for those who enjoy the heat!

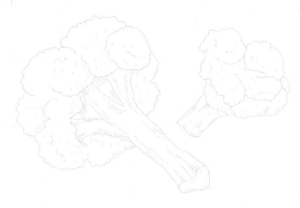

Chicken biryani with cauliflower rice

{ *SERVES* 2-3 }

The origins of this dish have been linked to Shah Jahan's queen, who inspired the Taj Mahal. It's said that she once visited army barracks and found the personnel undernourished. She asked the chef to prepare a special dish that provided balanced nutrition, and thus biryani was created!

700 g (1 lb 9 oz) skinless, boneless chicken thighs, cut in half

1 tablespoon coconut oil

1 brown onion, sliced

250 ml (9 fl oz/1 cup) coconut milk

1 cinnamon stick

2 cardamom pods

small handful coriander (cilantro) leaves, to serve

minted raita, to serve (see tip)

Marinade

1 teaspoon ground cumin

1 teaspoon ground coriander

1 teaspoon curry powder

1 teaspoon ground turmeric

1 × 2.5 cm (1 inch) piece ginger, peeled and grated

4 garlic cloves, crushed

1 green chilli, finely chopped

1 tablespoon lemon juice

Cauliflower rice

55 g (2 oz/1/4 cup) coconut oil

1 head cauliflower, riced (see page 75)

2 teaspoons ground cumin

1/4 teaspoon ground turmeric

handful coriander (cilantro) leaves, roughly chopped

handful mint, roughly chopped

sea salt and freshly ground black pepper, to taste

To make the marinade, mix all the ingredients in a large bowl.

Add the chicken pieces to the marinade, coat well then cover and marinate in the fridge for at least 1 hour.

Heat the coconut oil in a large frying pan over medium heat and fry the onion for 4-5 minutes, until translucent. Add the chicken and brown on both sides. Add the coconut milk, cinnamon stick and cardamom pods, and simmer for 15 minutes, or until the chicken is tender.

Meanwhile, make the cauliflower rice. Melt the oil in another large frying pan over medium heat. Add the cauliflower, mix in the spices, stir through the coriander and mint, and season with salt and pepper. Cook for 8-10 minutes, until soft.

Spoon the cauliflower rice into bowls and serve with the chicken in its sauce. Top with coriander and serve with minted raita.

SUPERCHARGED TIP

You can make a quick raita by mixing 1 chopped cucumber with 260 g (9¼ oz/1 cup) plain yoghurt and chopped mint to taste.

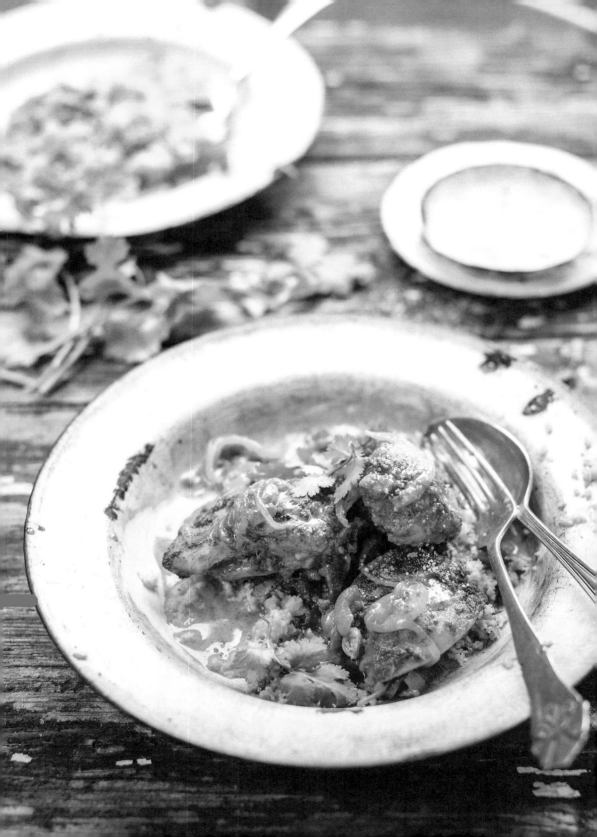

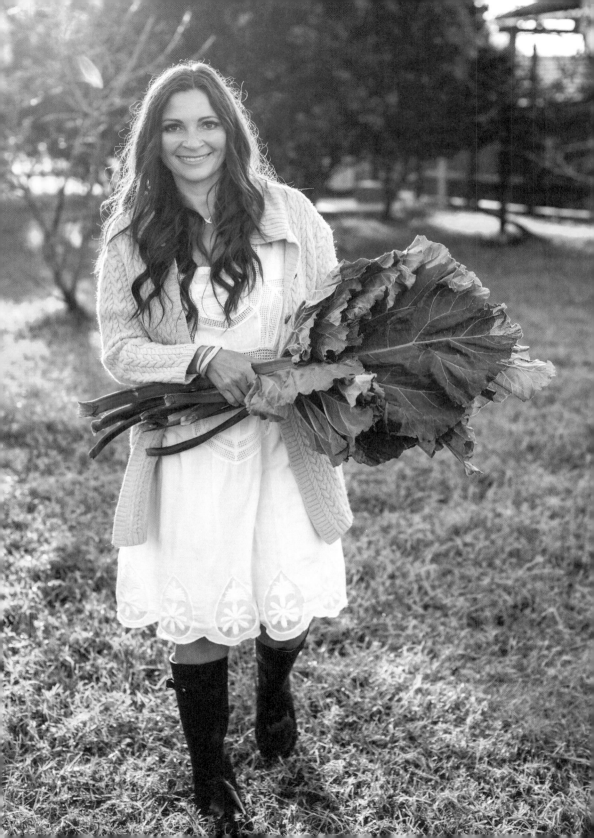

A cheerful heart

We live on an absolutely beautiful planet. While a million negative things regularly happen on our earth, I'm constantly in awe of the magical interplay between the order of the seasons and the cycles of nature; our potential for harmonious relationships with other humans and for nurturing our soil and our earth; and the immense blessing our planet brings us in return.

This is one of the reasons I started Supercharged Food. I'm astounded at the offering that can exist within even one herb that shoots from the ground, or one piece of fruit offered to us by a tree. I'm amazed by the medicinal properties that can exist within a piece of ginger, and how it seems almost meticulously designed specifically to heal the human body, whether it's to treat nausea or ease inflammatory conditions.

There's just so much to learn and to be grateful for in the process of growing, harvesting, gathering, preparing and enjoying the foods that the earth naturally provides for us, and loving the earth for its abundance is a good place to start.

My food philosophy has always been simple. Eating real, unmodified foods as close to the state that nature provides enables our bodies to function at their best. This means I run towards foods that are grown or reared naturally and are free from as much chemical intervention as possible.

For plants this means being grown in organic soils, free from synthetic fertilisers and sprays, where traditional methods of fertilisation are favoured. For animal products this means the animal has lived a life as nature would intend, free to roam in open fields and pastures, eating the grasses and bugs they naturally gravitate towards. It means avoiding eating animals that have been raised in the dark or other cruel conditions, or that have been fattened up on hormones, fed genetically modified seed meals or treated with antibiotics.

'In the depth of winter, I finally learned that within me there lay an invincible summer.'

—Albert Camus

I've been convinced throughout my own search for health and healing that every body is different and has different needs. It's our own responsibility to listen to our heart and steward our body through our lifestyle choices, ranging from movement, sleep and food right through to the emotional and spiritual factors that enable us to best maintain our health and find fulfilment. Along the way, I've learnt that:

- **THE GUT IS VITAL TO OUR OVERALL HEALTH:** More than 80 per cent of our immune system resides in our gut. Our bodies function best when we eat foods that support the healing of our gut lining, which may involve an elemental diet (easy-to-digest basics to give your gut a chance to heal; for more see my book *Heal Your Gut*) and intermittent fasting for a season. Smoothies, soups and gelatinous home-made broth-based meals are wonderful for the health of our gut lining. Probiotic and prebiotic foods are also important in creating the perfect environment for friendly bacteria to flourish.
- **WE SHOULD EAT ACCORDING TO OUR UNIQUE NEEDS:** I've been deeply impacted by the ancient healing art of Ayurveda. It's a whole-lifestyle approach that begins with determining your unique type, also known as a *dosha*. From there you can learn a host of lifestyle choices that best suit your emotional, physical, mental and spiritual needs. I love this philosophy, as it recognises that no one diet is perfect for everyone, and it empowers you to be the author of your own health based on the knowledge you've gained about your unique self. There's a multitude of information about Ayurveda and finding your *dosha* in my book *Eat Right for Your Shape*, which has all the information, tools and recipes you need to reap the benefits of the Ayurvedic philosophy.
- **WE SHOULD EAT WITH MINDFULNESS AND GRATITUDE:** Food that's considered, selected, prepared, served and enjoyed with genuine love and thankfulness will bless your body far more than you know. Eat slowly and not on the run. Taste, smell and experience all the sensations of your meals. Honour yourself by taking the time to sit down to eat. Chew your food and say thanks. Be grateful to the earth and to the divine blessing that food is.

A cheerful heart gives life to the body, and when it comes to food, balance and moderation are the key.

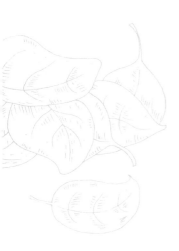

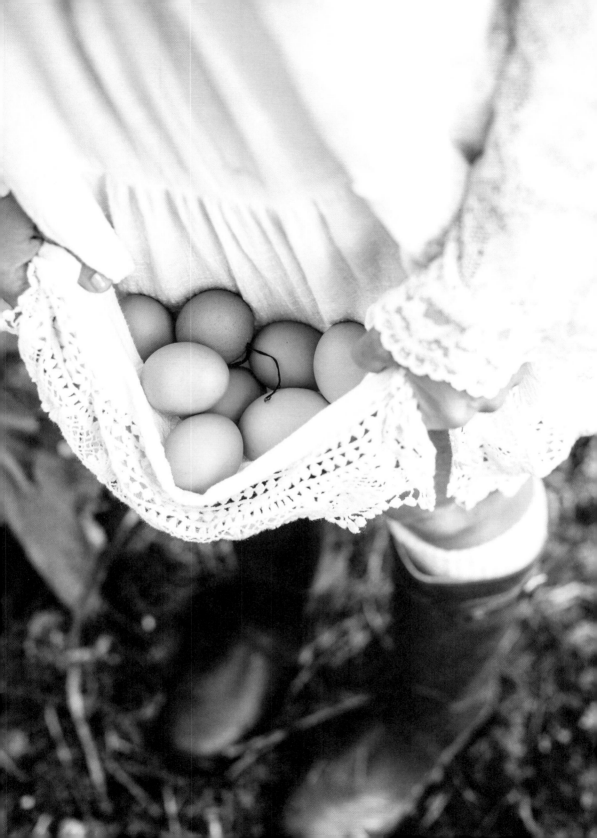

Balancing green smoothie

{ *SERVES* 1 }

A cooling bombshell and not your average green smoothie. This is a wonderful cleansing tonic for the body, especially with the addition of my Love Your Gut powder made from ground fossil shells, which will sweep gently through your tummy and remove impurities. You can find it on my website, superchargedfood.com.

½ avocado, peeled

2 kale leaves, spines removed, roughly chopped

125 ml (4 fl oz/½ cup) coconut milk

½ cucumber, peeled and chopped

125 ml (4 fl oz/½ cup) coconut water

1 teaspoon Love Your Gut Powder (optional)

Whiz all the ingredients in a high-speed blender or food processor until smooth. Taste and adjust the flavours, if necessary. Pour into a chilled drinking jar or glass and enjoy immediately.

Macacino

{ *SERVES* 2 }

500 ml (17 fl oz/2 cups) coconut milk

1 tablespoon coconut sugar or as needed

2 heaped tablespoons raw cacao powder

2 teaspoons maca powder

½ teaspoon vanilla powder

pinch of ground cinnamon

pinch of freshly grated nutmeg

pinch each of sea salt and freshly ground black pepper

Warm the coconut milk in a small saucepan over high heat then whisk in the remaining ingredients. Taste, adjust for sweetness and serve immediately.

SUPERCHARGED TIP
Pretty up the macacino with some edible flowers.

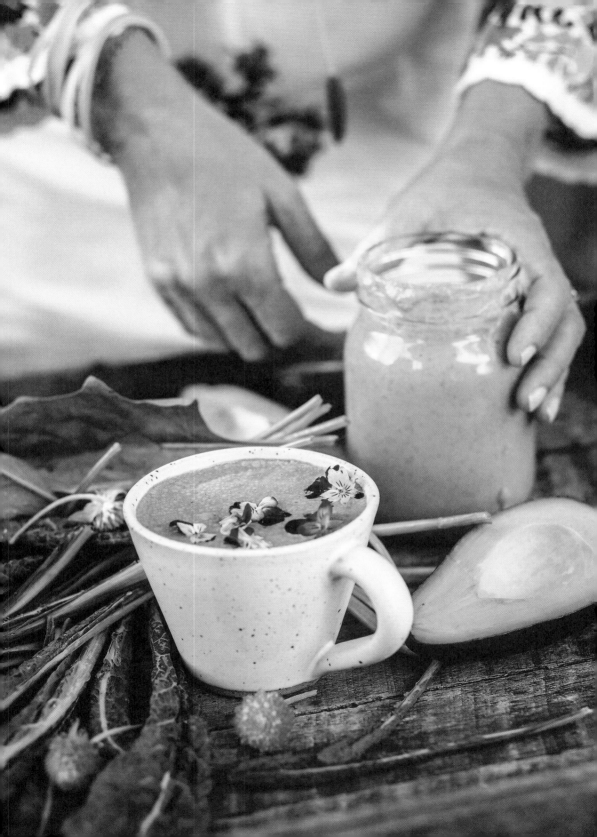

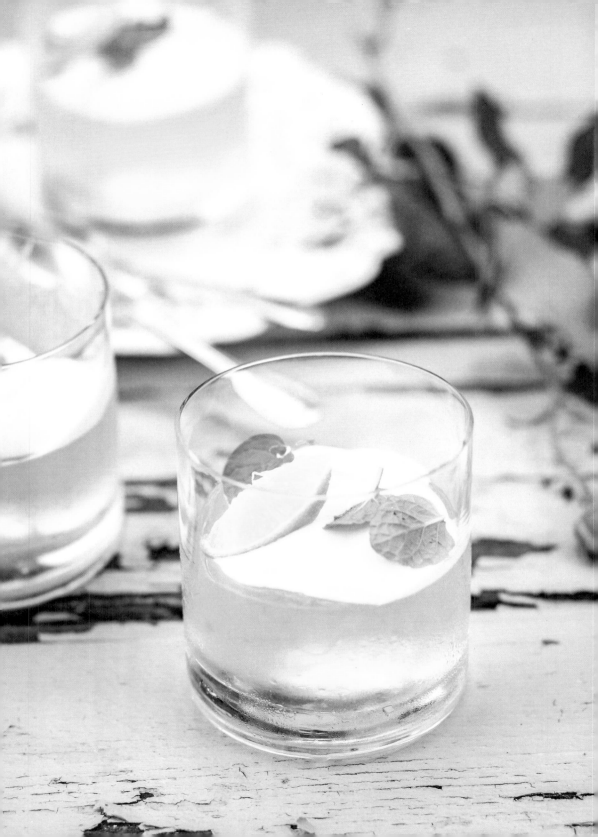

Aloe vera breakfast jelly with coconut 'yoghurt'

{ MAKES 4 DEPENDING ON SIZE OF JARS OR GLASSES }

A refreshing summertime breakfast or dessert, this healthy, all-natural jelly will be a delight for children and adults alike. The soothing properties of aloe vera decongest the lymphatic system and eliminate impurities. Aloe's bitter–cool quality is perfectly balanced, and its hydrating powers heal the skin from within by promoting the growth of collagen.

750 ml (26 fl oz/3 cups) aloe vera juice

1 tablespoon powdered gelatine

1 tablespoon lime juice

6 drops liquid stevia

small handful mint sprigs

1 teaspoon grated lime zest

Coconut 'Yoghurt' (page 195), mint leaves and lime wedges, to serve

Gently heat the aloe vera juice in a medium saucepan over medium–low heat until hot but not boiling, then add the gelatine and whisk until dissolved. Add the lime juice, stevia and mint, and continue to whisk while heating to a boil.

Remove from the heat, remove the mint sprigs and add the lime zest. Pour into glass jars or glasses, and chill in the fridge until set.

Serve topped with a dollop of coconut 'yoghurt', mint leaves and a lime wedge.

Turmeric and cardamom coconut lassi

{ *SERVES* 1-2 }

Enjoy this spicy twist on the traditional Indian lassi as the perfect afternoon snack when you're in the mood for a little sweetness. The aromatic chai flavours and the switch from dairy to creamy coconut yoghurt will provide a uniquely delectable experience.

250 ml (9 fl oz/1 cup) full-fat plain yoghurt or Coconut 'Yoghurt' (page 195)

1 frozen banana

250 ml (9 fl oz/1 cup) coconut water

1 teaspoon ground turmeric, plus extra to serve

pinch of ground cardamom

1/2 teaspoon ground cinnamon, plus extra to serve

1/2 teaspoon ground ginger

1/2 teaspoon vanilla powder

Whiz all the ingredients in a high-speed blender until smooth and creamy. Sprinkle with extra turmeric and cinnamon, and serve in large tall glasses.

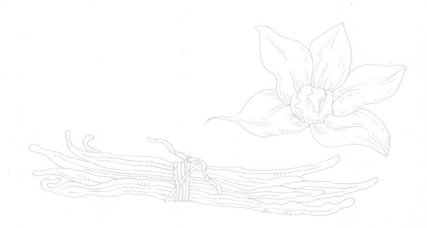

Poached chicken salad with blueberries and baked almond feta

{ SERVES 4 }

500 ml (17 fl oz/2 cups) filtered water

270 ml (9½ fl oz) coconut milk

2 large boneless, skinless chicken breasts

1 red onion, very thinly sliced

large handful coriander (cilantro) leaves, finely chopped

large handful mint leaves, chopped

2 handfuls parsley leaves, chopped

140 g (5 oz/1 cup) chopped roasted sweet potato

½ cup Baked Almond Feta (page 289), crumbled, or goat's cheese

2 tablespoons Almond, Pistachio and Hazelnut Dukkah (page 178)

Blueberry dressing

60 ml (2 fl oz/¼ cup) extra virgin olive oil

juice of ½ lemon

2 tablespoons apple cider vinegar

1 tablespoon sumac

1 teaspoon ground cumin

250 g (9 oz) blueberries

Mix the dressing ingredients in a small bowl.

Pour the water and coconut milk into a medium saucepan, place over medium heat and bring to the boil. Add the chicken, then reduce the heat to low and simmer for 9–12 minutes, until just cooked.

When ready to serve, slice or shred the chicken and arrange on a round platter with the herbs, sweet potato and feta. Sprinkle the dukkah over and serve.

Note: For a photo of this salad, see page 330.

Almond, pistachio and hazelnut dukkah

{ *MAKES ABOUT* 430 G [15¼ OZ / 2 CUPS] }

Use this dukkah as a balancing topping or as a crust on chicken or fish. You can fold it into your favourite dip, or sprinkle it on flatbreads, soups and baked vegetables.

110 g (3¾ oz/⅔ cup) almonds, chopped

70 g (2½ oz/½ cup) pistachio nut kernels, finely chopped

105 g (3¾ oz/⅔ cup) hazelnuts, chopped

75 g (2¾ oz/½ cup) sesame seeds

3 teaspoons coriander seeds

1 tablespoon cumin seeds

1 tablespoon paprika

1½ teaspoons ground turmeric

½ teaspoon freshly ground black pepper

1 teaspoon sea salt (optional)

Toast the nuts and sesame seeds in a dry heavy-based frying pan over medium heat, stirring often, until golden. Add the remaining ingredients and stir for about 1 minute, until aromatic. Allow to cool. Store in a glass jar with an airtight lid for up to 1 month.

Note: For a photo of this dukkah, see page 331.

Coconut sweet potato chips with avocado dipping sauce

{ *SERVES* 2-4 }

2 tablespoons melted coconut oil, plus extra for greasing

45 g (1½ oz/½ cup) desiccated coconut

2 teaspoons coconut flour

½ teaspoon ground turmeric

½ teaspoon paprika

½ teaspoon ground cinnamon

½ teaspoon chilli flakes (optional)

pinch each of sea salt and freshly ground black pepper

1 large sweet potato, peeled and cut into shoestring chips (fries)

Avocado dipping sauce

2 avocados, peeled

small handful coriander (cilantro) leaves, roughly chopped, plus extra for garnish

60 ml (2 fl oz/¼ cup) coconut cream

grated zest and juice of 1 lime

2 tablespoons olive oil

sea salt and freshly ground black pepper, to taste

Preheat the oven to 180°C (350°F) and grease a baking tray with a little extra coconut oil.

To make the avocado dipping sauce, in a medium bowl, mash the avocado with a fork, add the remaining ingredients and stir until well combined. Refrigerate until ready to use.

In a large bowl, mix together the coconut and coconut flour, spices, salt and pepper.

Massage the coconut oil into the sweet potato chips and roll them in the coconut mixture, using your hands to coat them well.

Spread the chips out evenly on the prepared baking tray and bake for 35-45 minutes, checking frequently to ensure they don't burn.

Serve hot with the dipping sauce on the side.

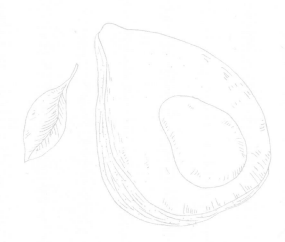

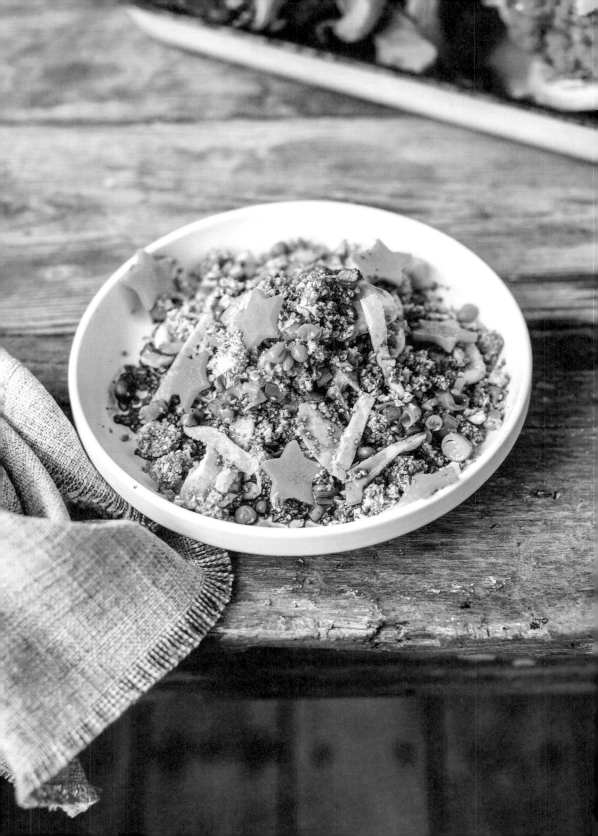

Cauliflower fried rice

{ *SERVES* 3–4 }

1 head cauliflower (I used an amazing purple variety here)

5 nitrate-free bacon rashers (slices), chopped

1 tablespoon sesame or coconut oil, plus extra as needed

3 eggs, whisked

large handful chopped spring onions (scallions)

1 tablespoon grated fresh ginger

3 garlic cloves, minced

500 g (1 lb 2 oz) boneless, skinless chicken breasts, chopped

90 g (3¼ oz/1 cup) sliced carrots (see tip)

140 g (5 oz/1 cup) frozen peas

6 anchovy fillets, chopped

2 tablespoons wheat-free tamari

1 tablespoon apple cider vinegar

1 tablespoon lime juice

handful coriander (cilantro) leaves, plus extra to serve (optional)

sesame seeds and lime wedges, to serve

Roughly chop the cauliflower into florets, then pulse in a food processor until it resembles rice. Set aside.

Heat a large wok over medium heat, then fry the bacon until brown and crispy. Set aside in a bowl.

Add a splash of sesame oil to the wok, then add the eggs, tilting the wok to spread them evenly, and fry, without stirring, until cooked through. Remove from the wok and roll up, then cut into slices.

Add a little more oil to the wok, increase the heat to high, then stir-fry the spring onion, ginger and garlic for 1 minute. Add the chicken and cook, stirring, to seal on all sides. Add the carrot and stir-fry until just tender, then turn out into a bowl with the cooked chicken.

Add a little more oil if needed, then add the cauliflower rice to the wok. Stir-fry for 3–5 minutes, until tender, then return all the cooked ingredients to the wok, along with the peas, anchovies, tamari, vinegar, lime juice and coriander, if using.

Serve warm, topped with sesame seeds and extra coriander, with lime wedges on the side.

SUPERCHARGED TIP

For a bit of fun, cut star shapes from some of the carrot.

Seafood chowder

{ SERVES 4 }

2 tablespoons olive oil

1 leek, pale part only, sliced

4 garlic cloves, chopped

3 tomatoes, chopped

1 tablespoon additive-free tomato paste (concentrated purée)

2 tablespoons apple cider vinegar

6 anchovy fillets, chopped

2 bay leaves

sea salt and freshly ground black pepper, to taste

400 g (14 oz) firm white fish fillets, cut into 5 cm (2 inch) pieces

1 litre (35 fl oz/4 cups) fish stock

270 ml (9½ fl oz) coconut milk

200 g (7 oz) raw prawns (shrimp), peeled and deveined

200 g (7 oz) mussels, scrubbed and beards removed

250 g (9 oz) cherry tomatoes

1 teaspoon grated lemon zest

juice of ½ lemon

15 g (½ oz/¼ cup) snipped chives

Heat the olive oil in a large saucepan over medium heat, then sauté the leek and garlic until softened. Add the tomato and cook for a further 5 minutes. Stir in the tomato paste, vinegar, anchovies and bay leaves, then return to a simmer. Season with salt and pepper.

Stir in the fish, stock and coconut milk, return to a simmer, then add the prawns, mussels, cherry tomatoes, and lemon zest and juice. Reduce the heat to low and simmer, covered, for about 5 minutes.

Transfer gently to bowls and serve garnished with the chives.

Garlic curry

{ *SERVES 2* }

I learnt this recipe at a cooking class in Sri Lanka, and it is unforgettable. Interestingly, the garlic is not super strong when cooked this way, and it tends to really sweeten up and get so soft and fragrant it literally melts in the mouth. Eat it with brown rice or your favourite substitute.

1 tablespoon sesame oil

½ teaspoon black mustard seeds

½ teaspoon fenugreek seeds

1 brown onion, sliced

6 curry leaves

1 small green chilli, seeded and chopped

2 teaspoons curry powder

¼ teaspoon asafoetida powder

½ teaspoon ground turmeric

5 garlic bulbs, cloves separated and peeled

sea salt, to taste

375 ml (13 fl oz/1½ cups) coconut milk, plus extra as needed

1 tablespoon rice malt syrup (optional)

Heat the sesame oil in a small heavy-based frying pan over medium heat. When the oil is shimmering, add the mustard seeds and fenugreek seeds, and fry until they start to pop. Add the onion and fry until golden, then add the curry leaves, chilli, curry powder, asafoetida and turmeric, stirring well. Stir in the garlic, salt and coconut milk.

Simmer, stirring occasionally, for 15 minutes, until the garlic is tender.

Top up with extra coconut milk if needed and add rice malt syrup to sweeten, if using.

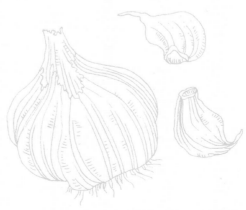

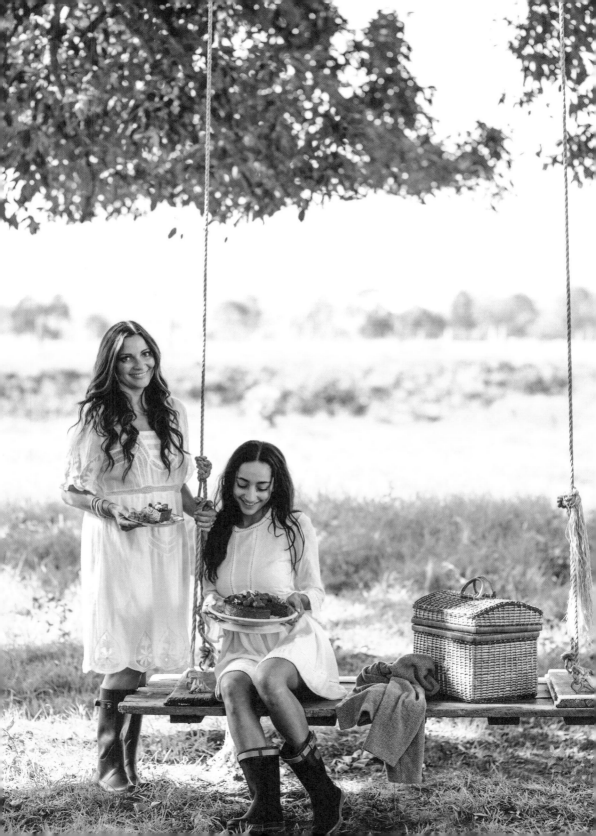

Feel-good food

Embracing a supercharged life and eating real food is about far more than just your own personal health. Although this embodiment of wellbeing helps us feel incredible, the best part is that we can have a positive impact on those around us.

When we eat in a healthy, balanced way our cells function optimally. Our body is operating at its peak, we can think clearly, we're full of energy, and our immune system is robust and able to defend us naturally from a range of minor illnesses that would otherwise slow us down. We have clarity in our thinking and our emotions are much less likely to be unstable. When we eat real food we feel good and we therefore extend joy and kindness into our relationships and other human interactions. We can fulfil our potential and pursue our life's work, whether that's parenting, a career, study or simple daily tasks that add up to make our big-picture story on this earth.

I believe that food isn't a separate or isolated compartment of my life that's significant only for supplying me with fuel and health. I truly see my choices surrounding food as having a dramatic effect on stewarding this earth and embracing the community around me. When we open our eyes to the power of our food choices and see the impact this daily interaction can have, it can be a soulful and spiritual experience. Read on, for some of my heart and soul recipes to cheer you and those you love.

'Good nutrition is important, and excellent health is a beautiful and necessary priority. But accessing the part of us that's indestructible, timeless, and that's born from love may be one of the biggest nutritional gifts we could ever give ourselves.' — *Marc David*

Chocolate matcha latte

{ *SERVES* 1 }

I love how this hot beverage just screams goodness. Who doesn't instantly feel good when consuming something so gorgeously green as matcha? Thankfully, even though my matcha latte is wildly healthy, you don't have to consume it purely for this reason. It's equally enjoyable for its warmth and sweetness.

1 teaspoon matcha tea powder

250 ml (9 fl oz/1 cup) coconut or almond milk

1 tablespoon rice malt syrup or stevia to taste

1 tablespoon cacao nibs (optional)

Put the matcha tea powder in a mug.

Gently warm the coconut milk and rice malt syrup in a small saucepan over low heat, then whisk until frothy. Pour onto the matcha powder and stir vigorously until blended. Top with the cacao nibs, if using, and enjoy the green goodness.

SUPERCHARGED TIP

If you want to pretty things up, scatter over a few edible flowers, such as chamomile.

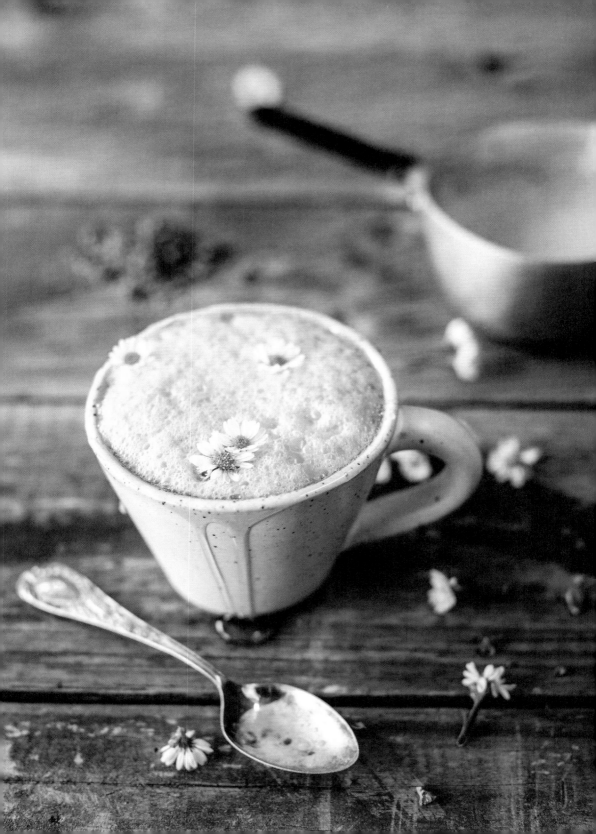

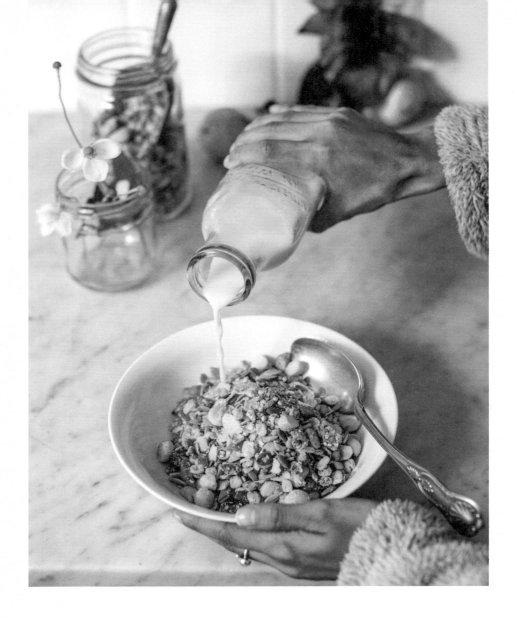

Apricot and macadamia granola

{ *SERVES* 8 }

Making a big batch of nutritious granola is one of the best ways to ensure you have a healthy breakfast treat on hand every day. This banging formulation will lend you a load of energy for tackling your to-do list! Make the most of a batch-cooking day by quadrupling the recipe and storing the excess in your pantry.

130 g (4½ oz/1 cup) roughly chopped dried apricots

155 g (5½ oz/1 cup) macadamia nuts, halved

200 g (7 oz/1²/₃ cups) quinoa flakes

200 g (7 oz/3⅓ cups) brown rice flakes

95 g (3¼ oz/1 cup) flaked almonds

50 g (1¾ oz/¼ cup) buckwheat groats

105 g (3¾ oz/²/₃ cup) pepitas (pumpkin seeds)

50 g (1¾ oz/⅓ cup) sesame seeds

105 g (3¾ oz/²/₃ cup) sunflower seeds

50 g (1¾ oz/⅓ cup) linseeds (flaxseeds)

1 teaspoon freshly grated nutmeg

1 teaspoon ground cinnamon

125 ml (4 fl oz/½ cup) caramelised apple cider vinegar (below)

2 teaspoons vanilla powder or alcohol-free vanilla extract

almond milk, to serve

Caramelised apple cider vinegar

250 ml (9 fl oz/1 cup) apple cider vinegar

2 tablespoons rice malt syrup or your sweetener of choice

To make the caramelised apple cider vinegar, heat the vinegar and syrup in a small saucepan over medium heat. Bring to the boil and continue boiling until reduced by half. Remove from the heat and allow to cool.

Preheat the oven to 180°C (350°F) and line a large baking tray with baking paper.

Combine all the granola ingredients except the vinegar, vanilla and almond milk in a large bowl. Mix thoroughly. Stir in the caramelised apple cider vinegar and vanilla.

Spread out on the prepared baking tray and bake on the middle shelf of the oven for 25–30 minutes, stirring after 20 minutes and adjusting the flavours as needed.

Allow to cool, then store in an airtight container in the pantry for up to 4 weeks.

Apricot muesli bars

{ *MAKES* 8 }

Once you have the granola ready, it takes just minutes to create these delicious muesli bars. They're perfect for a breakfast on the run, to take to work for morning tea, or as an afternoon snack for the kids.

75 g (2¾ oz/¾ cup) gluten-free rolled (porridge) oats

¼ quantity Apricot and Macadamia Granola (page 188)

75 g (2¾ oz/½ cup) dried cranberries

180 g (6¼ oz/½ cup) rice malt syrup

Preheat the oven to 180°C (350°F) and line a 20 cm (8 inch) square cake tin with baking paper.

Optional step: you can toast the oats in the oven (spread out on a baking tray) for 15–20 minutes, until slightly golden. Otherwise, leave them uncooked.

Process the cranberries in a food processor until sticky.

Combine all the ingredients in a medium bowl and stir with a wooden spoon until well mixed.

Push the mixture into the prepared tin and bake on the middle shelf of the oven for 15 minutes, or until slightly crisp (see tip).

Cool, then cut into eight bars. Store in an airtight container in the fridge for up to 2 weeks.

SUPERCHARGED TIP

Instead of baking the mixture, you can leave it raw, push it into a square dish and allow to set in the fridge for 30 minutes. Cut into eight bars and store in an airtight container in the fridge for up to 2 weeks.

Teff pancakes two ways: sweet and savoury!

Teff, an Ethiopian staple, is one of the smallest gluten-free grains in the world, about the size of a poppy seed. It's rich in calcium and essential amino acids. Try teff pancakes sweet, with berries, or savoury, with eggs and salmon (page 192).

Basic teff pancakes

{ *MAKES* 12 }

180 g (6¼ oz/2¼ cups) teff flour

1 tablespoon gluten-free baking powder

1 tablespoon arrowroot powder

½ teaspoon sea salt

2 tablespoons coconut oil

1 egg, whisked

625 ml (21½ fl oz/2½ cups) almond milk, plus extra as needed

1 teaspoon vanilla powder

1 teaspoon ground cinnamon

Heat a large frying pan over medium heat.

Combine the teff flour, baking powder, arrowroot powder and salt in a large bowl. Add the remaining ingredients and stir until well combined, adding more almond milk if necessary to obtain the desired pouring consistency.

Working in batches, add 60 ml (2 fl oz/¼ cup) dollops of the batter to the pan. Cook until bubbles form on the surface, then turn over and cook the other side. Repeat with the remaining batter.

Teff pancakes with rice malt syrup and berries

{ *SERVES* 2 }

1 quantity Teff Pancakes (above)

2 tablespoons rice malt syrup

mixed berries, to serve

Drizzle the rice malt syrup over the hot pancakes and tumble on the fresh berries. >

Teff pancakes with smoked salmon, pesto and poached eggs

{ *SERVES* 2 }

dash of apple cider vinegar

4 large eggs

½ quantity Teff Pancakes (page 191)

2 smoked salmon slices

1 quantity Spinach and Hazelnut Pesto (page 229)

1 lemon, halved

Hummus dressing

60 ml (2 fl oz/¼ cup) coconut milk

55 g (2 oz/¼ cup) hummus

2 tablespoons tahini

1 teaspoon lemon zest

sea salt, to taste

splash of sesame oil (optional)

To make the hummus dressing, combine all the ingredients in a small bowl and stir well.

Bring a medium saucepan of water to a simmer, add the vinegar and poach the eggs to your liking. Place two or three teff pancakes on each plate and top with a slice of salmon, two eggs and a dollop of pesto.

Serve with lemon halves for squeezing and the hummus dressing.

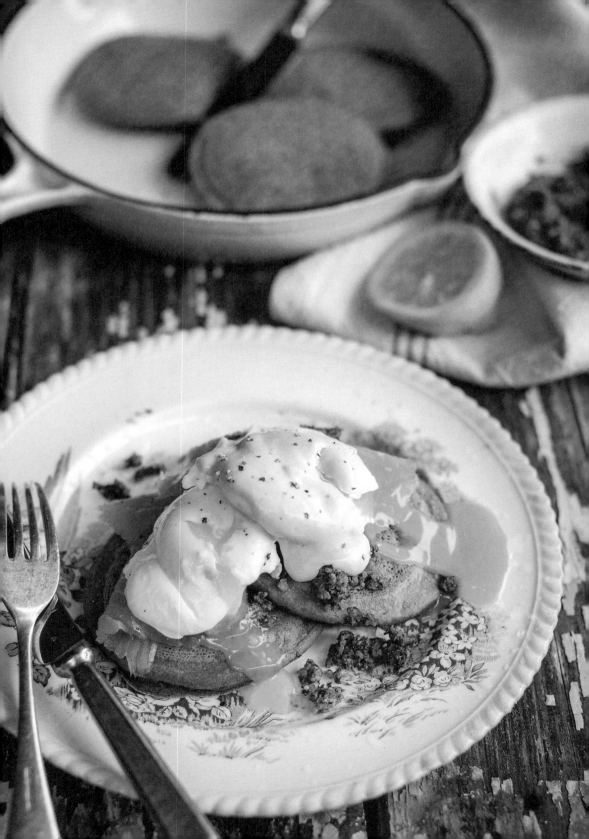

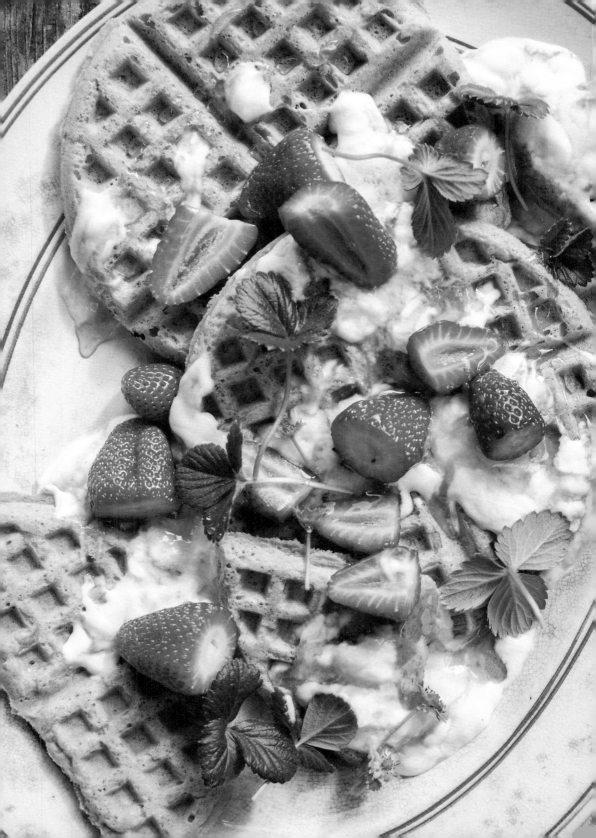

Waffles with fresh strawberries and coconut 'yoghurt'

{ *SERVES* 4 }

I love what joy a waffle-maker can bring to my life. It's amazing how a few simple ingredients can be pressed into that magical latticed shape and the next moment you're enjoying the tastiest and most decadent treat. These sweet darlings are topped with juicy strawberries and coconut yoghurt, but they're also great with nut butter. Good fun for little kids and big kids alike.

165 g (5¾ oz/1½ cups) oat flour

2 teaspoons gluten-free baking powder

½ teaspoon sea salt

½ teaspoon ground cinnamon

185 ml (6 fl oz/¾ cup) coconut milk

100 g (3½ oz) unsalted butter or coconut oil, melted

2 large eggs

½ teaspoon stevia powder or 2 tablespoons rice malt syrup

1 teaspoon alcohol-free vanilla extract

1 teaspoon apple cider vinegar

rice malt syrup, strawberries and strawberry leaves and young fruit (optional), to serve

Coconut 'yoghurt'

170 g (6 oz/2 cups) fresh young Thai coconut meat (see tip)

125 ml (4 fl oz/½ cup) coconut water

2 teaspoons lemon juice

pinch of fine sea salt

½ teaspoon stevia powder or your sweetener of choice (optional)

To make the coconut yoghurt, whiz all the ingredients in a blender until smooth and creamy. Spoon the yoghurt into an airtight container and chill in the fridge.

In a medium bowl, combine the oat flour, baking powder, salt and cinnamon. In a separate bowl, whisk together the coconut milk, butter, eggs, stevia, vanilla and apple cider vinegar. Pour the wet ingredients into the dry and stir until well combined. Set the batter aside for 10 minutes to thicken.

Heat the waffle maker, spoon in a portion of batter and cook until golden. Leave on a wire rack to cool slightly and crisp up while repeating the process with the remaining batter.

Serve topped with coconut 'yoghurt', rice malt syrup, strawberries and strawberry leaves and young fruit, if using.

SUPERCHARGED TIP

Young coconut meat has a softer, more gelatinous texture and comes from the smooth, green coconut rather than the hairy brown mature coconut.

Cranberry, fig and almond loaf with goat's cheese and avocado

{ MAKES 9 x 30 CM [3½ x 12 INCH] LOAF }

butter, for greasing, plus extra to serve (optional)

200 g (7 oz/2 cups) almond meal, plus extra for dusting

pinch of sea salt

¼ teaspoon gluten-free baking powder

2 ripe bananas, mashed

60 ml (2 fl oz/¼ cup) coconut milk

2 large eggs

95 g (3¼ oz/½ cup) dried figs, chopped

75 g (2¾ oz/½ cup) dried cranberries

1 teaspoon orange zest

1 teaspoon vanilla powder

140 g (5 oz/1 cup) mixed chopped nuts and seeds (e.g. slivered almonds, pistachio nut kernels, walnuts, hazelnuts, sunflower seeds, pepitas/pumpkin seeds), plus extra to decorate

avocado or butter and goat's cheese, to serve (optional)

Preheat the oven to 180°C (350°F). Grease a 9 × 30 cm (3½ × 12 inch) loaf (bar) tin with butter and line it with baking paper.

In a medium bowl, combine the almond meal, salt and baking powder, and mix well. In a separate bowl, combine the banana, coconut milk and eggs, and whisk until smooth. Fold the dry ingredients into the wet ingredients until thoroughly combined. Fold in the figs, cranberries, orange zest, vanilla, nuts and seeds.

Spoon the mixture into the prepared tin and sprinkle with the extra nuts and seeds. Bake for 40 minutes, or until a knife inserted into the centre comes out clean. Cool the loaf in the tin for 1 hour.

For breakfast, serve toasted and smothered with avocado or butter and goat's cheese.

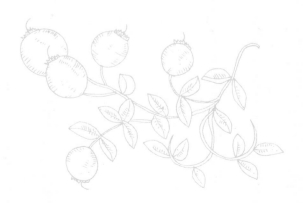

Chicken schnitzel with parsnip mash

{ *SERVES* 4 }

The crispy golden crunch of a schnitzel is a fulfilling memory for many, but unfortunately this Viennese dish is often spoiled by poor-quality ingredients. Redeem the illustrious schnitzel and prepare for your diners to be amazed.

100 g (3½ oz/1 cup) almond meal

120 g (4¼ oz/1 cup) coconut flour

1 teaspoon paprika

sea salt and freshly ground black pepper, to taste

3 eggs

65 g (2¼ oz/½ cup) arrowroot or tapioca flour

4 boneless, skinless chicken breasts, sliced in half crossways

2 tablespoons coconut oil

green leafy salad, to serve

Parsnip mash

2 tablespoons extra virgin olive oil

1 tablespoon filtered water, plus extra, boiling, as needed

1 brown onion, diced

8 parsnips, peeled and roughly chopped

1 teaspoon dried thyme

1 teaspoon dried oregano

sea salt and freshly ground black pepper, to taste

To make the mash, heat half the olive oil with the water in a large saucepan over medium heat. Add the onion and sauté for 3–4 minutes, until translucent. Add the parsnips, then enough boiling water to cover. Stir in the herbs, salt and pepper, then bring to the boil. Reduce the heat to low and simmer for 25 minutes, or until the parsnips are soft.

Carefully pour the parsnip cooking liquid into a jar (refrigerate and use as a vegetable stock, or drink it as a nourishing beverage straight away), leaving just a little bit in the pan. Add the remaining oil to the parsnips and purée using a hand-held blender. Set aside and keep warm.

To make the schnitzels, take three shallow bowls. Mix the almond meal, coconut flour, paprika, salt and pepper in one bowl. Whisk the eggs in the second and place the arrowroot flour in the third.

Pound the chicken to uniform thickness using a rolling pin or mallet. (The tidiest way to do this is in a snaplock bag with the air pushed out.) Coat each piece of chicken in the arrowroot flour, then the egg, then the almond mixture. Make sure each piece is evenly coated.

Heat half the coconut oil in a large frying pan over medium–high heat. Fry the chicken in two batches for 4–5 minutes on each side, adding the remaining oil for the second batch.

Serve the chicken and mash with a green salad.

Sesame-crusted fish and lotus chips

{ *SERVES* 4 }

4 skinless firm white fish fillets

sea salt and freshly ground
  black pepper, to taste

145 g (5 oz/1 cup) sesame seeds,
  toasted

60 ml (2 fl oz/¼ cup)
  macadamia oil

handful mint or coriander
  (cilantro) leaves

lime halves, to serve

Cumin-spiced Lotus Root Chips
  (page 120), to serve

Hummus Dressing (page 192),
  to serve (optional)

Preheat the oven to 180°C (350°F).

Heat a large heavy-based frying pan over
medium heat.

Season the fish fillets with salt and pepper. Put
the sesame seeds on a plate, then press the
fillets onto the seeds, patting them on to coat
as well as possible on both sides.

Add the macadamia oil to the pan and heat
until it shimmers. Add the fillets and fry for
2–3 minutes, then carefully turn them over
and fry on the other side for 1–2 minutes,
until cooked through.

Serve the fish with mint or coriander, lime
halves and lotus chips. Offer the hummus
dressing, if using, on the side.

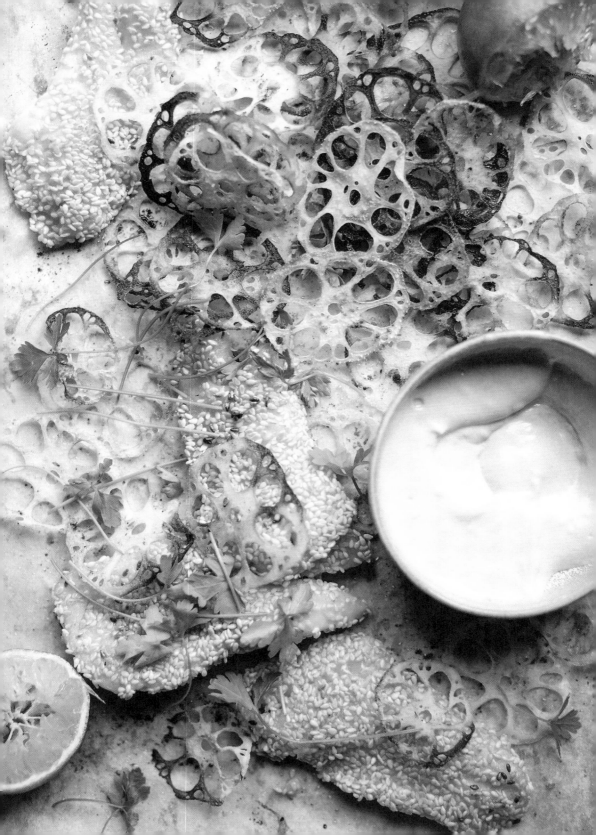

Egg and wild mushroom tart

{ *SERVES 6* }

Crust

300 g (10½ oz/3 cups) almond meal

pinch of sea salt

1½ teaspoons bicarbonate of soda (baking soda)

1 teaspoon dried rosemary

125 ml (4 fl oz/½ cup) extra virgin olive oil or melted butter

2 tablespoons cold filtered water

Filling

25 g (1 oz) butter or 1 tablespoon olive oil

1 French shallot, finely chopped

2 garlic cloves, finely chopped

300 g (10½ oz) mixed mushrooms, chopped

handful parsley, chopped

sea salt and freshly ground black pepper, to taste

3 eggs

400 ml (14 fl oz) coconut milk

2 tablespoons nutritional yeast flakes

Preheat the oven to 180°C (350°F) and lightly grease a 22 cm (8½ inch) flan (tart) tin.

To make the crust, combine the almond meal, salt, bicarbonate of soda and rosemary in a large bowl and mix well.

In a separate bowl, whisk the olive oil with half the water. Stir the olive oil and water into the dry ingredients and mix well to combine. If the mixture is too dry, add more water. Push into the base and sides of the prepared tin. Bake for 10 minutes.

Meanwhile, make the filling. Heat a large frying pan over medium heat, then add the butter and fry the shallot, garlic and mushrooms for 5 minutes, or until there is no liquid left in the pan. Add the parsley and season with salt and pepper.

While the mushrooms are cooking, whisk the eggs, coconut milk and yeast flakes in a medium bowl.

Allow the crust to cool slightly before spooning in the mushroom mixture, then pour the egg mixture over.

Bake for 25–35 minutes, until the crust is golden and the filling is set.

Note: For a photo of this tart, see page 337.

SUPERCHARGED TIP
This tart is lovely topped with fresh basil leaves.

Chicken, mushroom and thyme quinoa risotto

{ *SERVES* 4 }

1.5 litres (52 fl oz/6 cups) chicken stock

2 boneless, skinless chicken breasts, cut into strips

2 tablespoons extra virgin olive oil, plus extra for drizzling

1 brown onion, finely chopped

2 garlic cloves, sliced

200 g (7 oz) Swiss brown mushrooms, thinly sliced

200 g (7 oz/1 cup) white quinoa, thoroughly rinsed and drained

grated zest of 1 lemon

4 thyme sprigs, leaves picked

50 g (1³/₄ oz) rocket (arugula), shredded

sea salt and freshly ground black pepper, to taste

20 g (³/₄ oz/¹/₄ cup) nutritional yeast flakes

Bring the stock to the boil in a large saucepan over medium heat, then add the chicken and simmer for 7–8 minutes. Remove the chicken using tongs, then slice and set aside.

Meanwhile, heat the olive oil in a separate large saucepan over medium heat and sauté the onion, garlic and mushrooms for 1–2 minutes. Stir in the quinoa, lemon zest and thyme. Add half the stock and bring to the boil, then reduce the heat to low and simmer, covered, for 15 minutes, stirring frequently. Add the chicken pieces and cook, stirring for a further 5–7 minutes, adding ladlefuls of the remaining stock as each one is absorbed (see tip).

When the quinoa is cooked, remove from the heat, stir in the rocket, season with salt and pepper, and sprinkle the yeast flakes over.

Serve with a drizzle of extra olive oil.

SUPERCHARGED TIP

As with all risottos, the trick with this recipe is to add the stock gradually to ensure a beautiful, oozy consistency.

Meatloaf with sweet lemon thyme roasted carrots

{ *MAKES 9 x 30 CM [3½ x 12 INCH] LOAF OR 12 SLICES* }

1 kg (2 lb 4 oz) minced (ground) beef

150 g (5½ oz/1½ cups) almond meal

1 brown onion, grated

1 carrot, grated

1 zucchini (courgette), grated

2 heaped tablespoons additive-free tomato paste (concentrated purée)

2 tablespoons chopped flat-leaf (Italian) parsley leaves

1 large egg, lightly beaten

sea salt and freshly ground black pepper, to taste

350 g (12 oz) green beans, steamed

Sweet Lemon Thyme Roasted Carrots (page 93) and a microherb salad, to serve

Preheat the oven to 180°C (350°F) and line a baking tray or a bar (loaf) tin with baking paper.

Combine the minced beef, almond meal, onion, carrot, zucchini, tomato paste, parsley and egg in a large bowl. Season with salt and pepper, and mix well using clean hands. Shape the mixture into a rectangular loaf on the prepared baking tray or spoon into the loaf tin and smooth the top.

Bake for 25–30 minutes or until firm. Remove from the oven and drain off the excess fat.

Serve with the steamed beans, sweet lemon thyme roasted carrots and microherb salad.

SUPERCHARGED TIP

Not sure what to do with the left-over meatloaf? Try my delicious Meatloaf Laksa with Rice Noodles (page 165). Sorted!

Meat-lover's pizza with cauliflower crust

{ *SERVES* 4 }

olive oil for greasing (optional) and frying

500 g (1 lb 2 oz) beef, cut into strips

125 g (4½ oz/½ cup) additive-free tomato paste (concentrated purée)

1 large cauliflower pizza base (below)

125 g (4½ oz/½ cup) Cashew and Basil Pesto (page 228)

1 brown onion, diced

½ green capsicum (pepper), seeded and diced

2 handfuls rocket (arugula) or baby English spinach leaves

80 g (2¾ oz/1 cup) nutritional yeast flakes or mozzarella cheese, grated

Shoestring Sweet Potato Fries (page 125), to serve

Cauliflower pizza base

300 g (10½ oz/1 cup) grated cauliflower, steamed

1 egg

100 g (3½ oz/1 cup) almond meal

1–2 garlic cloves, finely chopped

pinch of caraway seeds

40 g (1½ oz/½ cup) nutritional yeast flakes

1½ teaspoons dried Italian herbs

1½ teaspoons dried parsley

Preheat the oven to 230°C (450°F). Grease a baking tray with olive oil or line it with baking paper.

To make the pizza base, combine the cauliflower, egg, almond meal, garlic, caraway seeds and yeast flakes in a bowl. Spoon the mixture onto the prepared baking tray and press into a square of uniform thickness. Sprinkle the herbs over. Bake for 12–15 minutes, until firm and browned. Remove from the oven and allow the base to cool slightly.

Meanwhile, heat a little olive oil in a medium frying pan over high heat, then sauté the beef strips in two batches until browned. Set aside.

Spread the tomato paste over the pizza base, then top with the pesto, onion, capsicum, beef and rocket, and sprinkle on the yeast flakes. Return to the oven for a further 5–10 minutes.

Serve with the sweet potato fries.

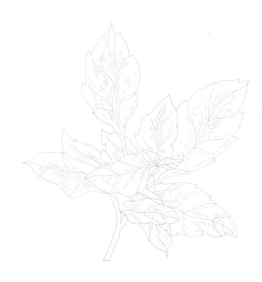

Peanut butter mousse

{ SERVES 2 }

270 ml (9½ fl oz) full-fat
  coconut cream, refrigerated
  overnight to thicken

70 g (2½ oz/¼ cup) natural
  peanut butter

10 drops liquid stevia or
  1 tablespoon rice malt syrup

½ teaspoon alcohol-free vanilla
  extract

½ teaspoon raw cacao powder

pinch of sea salt

desiccated coconut, cacao nibs
  and/or salted nuts, roughly
  chopped, to serve

edible flowers, to serve
  (optional)

Drain off the small amount of liquid on top of
the coconut cream and transfer the remainder
to a medium bowl. Add the peanut butter,
stevia, vanilla, cacao powder and salt, then
beat with an electric mixer, until the mixture
resembles whipped cream.

Spoon the mousse into small serving glasses,
top with desiccated coconut, cacao nibs
and/or nuts, and garnish with edible flowers,
if using.

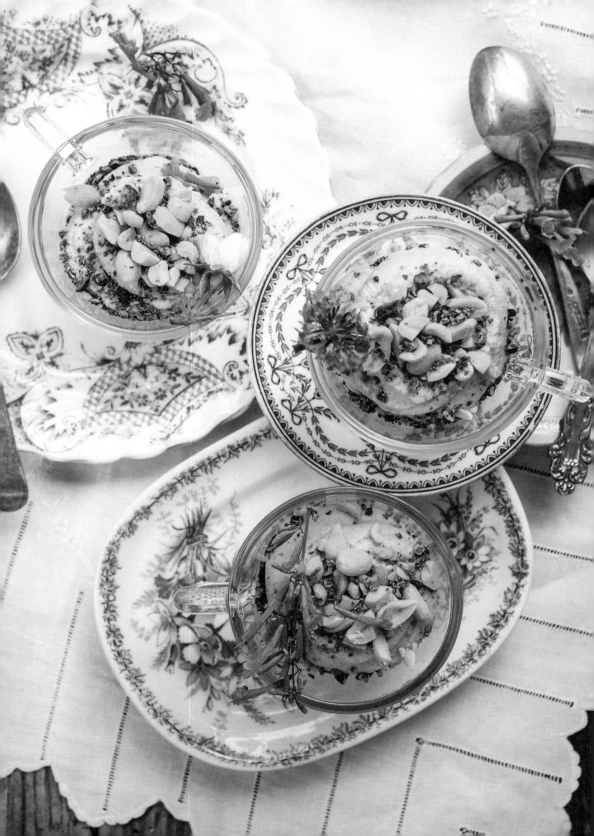

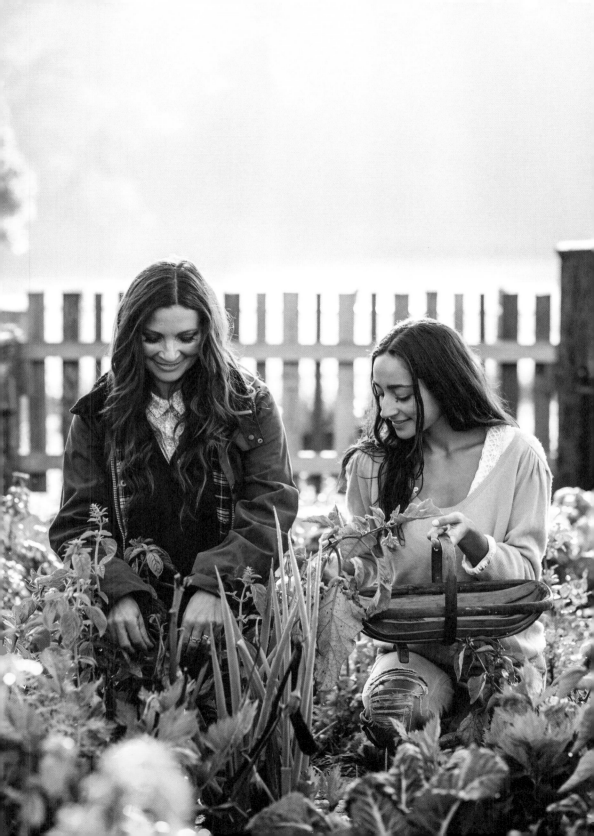

Starting in your own backyard

Those of you who've tasted a sun-sweetened strawberry fresh off the plant and still warm from the garden will agree when I say there's nothing quite like its unique taste. Freshly picked, with its tickly external texture and intense burst of flavour that tangs your tastebuds and stains your lips with a beautiful ruby-red tint, the strawberry is one of nature's finest ingredients, and it beats the taste of anything you'll find on the supermarket shelves.

Only a few generations ago, much of our food was growing in gardens only hours before it was served up at the family dinner table. The benefits of growing your own food are enormous, from its taste right through to its economic and environmental impacts.

THE EDIBLE GARDEN

If you're in a position to grow your own food (and you don't already), then why not start by planting a few seeds in your own backyard? Once fruits and vegetables are picked or harvested, their nutrients immediately begin to disappear and will keep doing so until the product is consumed, so you can be sure your home-grown produce will be flavour-packed and filled with vital nutrients. It's also more economical to eat home-grown fruit and veg, and if you have an abundance you can freeze it for the coming months – or give it to your neighbours and friends.

When food is out of season but still available on your local supermarket shelves, it's been grown interstate, overseas or in an artificial environment such as a greenhouse and transported via roads, sea or air so you can put it on your plate. This can mean the food spending weeks or months in transit. Rotting is prevented by harvesting the product before it's fully ripe, which also means the food hasn't developed its full nutrient or flavour potential. There's also the problem of its carbon footprint and the impact on our environment.

The intense, vibrant colours of home-grown produce, ripened by nothing other than the air and the sun, should be a focal point on the kitchen table.

> 'We have not inherited the earth from our fathers,
> we are borrowing it from our children.'
> – Lester R. Brown, *Building a Sustainable Society*

I've created a small vegetable patch in my garden beginning with a few key ingredients, including the following gems.

Strawberries

My strawberries are flourishing. I began with small plants (seedlings) I picked up at a local nursery. They require full sun to grow and moist, well-drained soil. Never place strawberries in the fridge, because the low temperatures steal their fragrance and flavour, and anything you leave in the fridge with them can quickly absorb their flavour. Washing them can make them go a bit mushy, so I generally wipe mine with damp paper towel. I use strawberries to make granita, ice cream and smoothies. A beautiful salad combo is strawberry, kale, avocado and pistachio, to which I usually add a simple extra virgin olive oil and lemon dressing. In Australia, strawberries have two seasons, summer and winter. In summer the strawberries come from New South Wales and Victoria, and in winter they are grown in Queensland.

Cucumbers

I stumbled upon a small cucumber plant at my local nursery and was told they're a good all-round grower. I admit the fruit it produces is a bit knobbly to look at, but what they lack in beauty they make up for with their beautiful taste. They're planted along the side of my house, where I grow jasmine on a wire trellis. To support my cucumbers I constructed a simple wigwam-type trellis from bamboo canes, because they're vines and like to do a spot of climbing – and, importantly, I wanted to conserve space.

This area gets the sun and I've put in an automatic watering system, as cucumbers get thirsty and can be bitter with insufficient moisture. It's best to harvest cucumbers within 8–10 weeks and to cut the fruit off with secateurs or a sharp knife. In my frost-free climate, as I observe the seasons shifting before my eyes, the humble cucumber is a seasonal mainstay, continuing to transition well from month to month throughout the changing year.

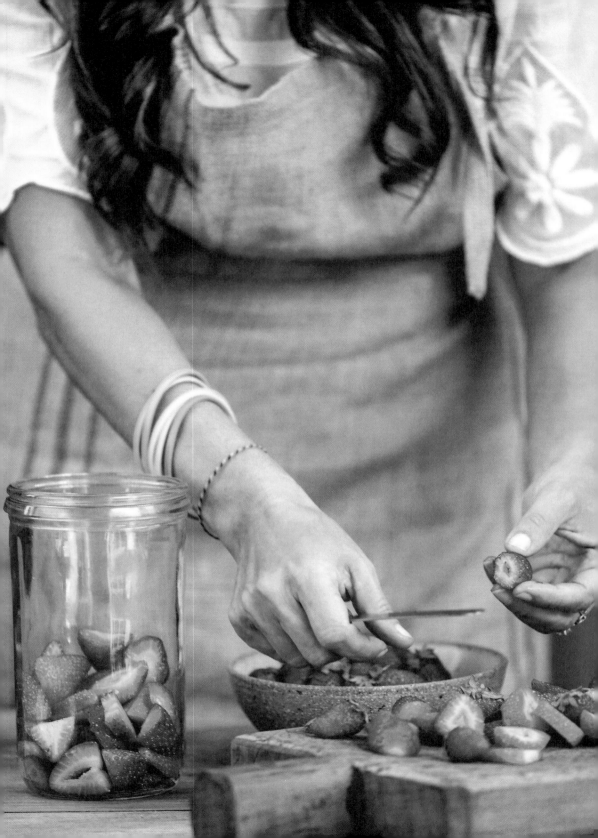

I love cucumbers in juices, salads and sandwiches, and often whiz up cucumber noodles (coodles) to enjoy with a yummy basil and cashew pesto. Cucumbers are the perfect summer food: refreshing and mellow, sweet and perfectly light. Even nibbling on them as a snack is a powerful thirst-quencher. In summer I like to cut a few slices and add them to mineral water for a refreshing drink. Keep them on the top shelf of your fridge, as being too cold leads to water-soaked areas, pitting and accelerated decay. Cucumber ages other fruit, so don't store these guys next to other fruit. They can also dehydrate easily.

Tomatoes

I love that tomatoes can be found in beautiful sunny shades of ruby-red and orange, purple and even black, and in many different sizes, shapes and flavours. My roma (plum) tomatoes are snuggled in a hanging basket, nestled in the warmth under cover. Roma is the traditional Italian egg-shaped tomato that goes well in salads, oven-roasted with herbs or made into a paste. Toms love warmth, and you can even grow them indoors if you don't have a garden. I use them regularly in my salads and when I make my special lamb bolognese.

These rosy bundles of sumptuousness can be sauced, pasta-ised, baked, slow-roasted, used raw, made into soups, squished into dips and even blended into sorbets and puddings. I find that slow-roasting tomatoes is a simple yet utterly transformative process with sweet and delicious results. I generally roast my romas or vine-ripened cherry tomatoes in a 150°C (300°F) oven with a drizzle of extra virgin olive oil, some apple cider vinegar and rosemary for 1 hour, and they come out all caramelised and delicious.

Stuffed tomatoes are an exotic way to incorporate a host of delicious in-season vegetables into one glorious mouthful. You could accompany stuffed tomatoes with a crunchy salad or have them as a side dish to your main.

To ripen tomatoes, put them in a brown paper bag and leave them at room temperature until they're ready, usually within a day or two. Store ripe whole tomatoes in a cool place and they should stay fresh for up to five days. Once you've cut tomatoes, though, the best place to store them is in the fridge.

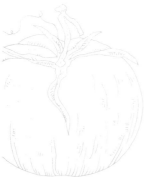

HERBS

Herbs are a dream come true in the kitchen; there's hardly a dish that doesn't benefit from including them. If expensive supermarket herbs are financially unsustainable, it's very easy to grow your own – you don't need a green thumb or heaps of space. A little herb garden really is a wonderful thing; all herbs require is some sunshine, good soil that drains well, regular watering, and a little love and attention. They're much easier to grow than house plants and a good money-saving hobby. You can grow them in pots very successfully, but as they grow and spread out they do prefer to be planted in the ground.

Although I have a small backyard, I've built a herb wall in my vegetable garden, complete with a composting unit for recycling any waste. Spending time in the garden each morning before work allows me to breathe in the unmistakable scents of fresh basil and rosemary wafting up into my nostrils as I pick the herbs I'm going to be using for the day.

Finding the best spot in your garden or on your windowsill is the first step. Most herbs like full sun or at least filtered light. If you're growing them in a container they can sit on a sunny deck or patio in clay pots, or up on a wall on a wire frame.

When herbs outgrow their pots, you can transfer them to larger ones or upcycle whatever you have on hand, such as old tubs or containers, adding drainage holes if necessary. Fill your pots with good potting soil and use organic fertiliser. When you're planting your herbs, just make sure you leave sufficient space between them to allow for growth, and also wet the soil well with a watering can or hose with a spray attachment.

If you're planting from smaller seedlings, tip the pots upside down and tap the bottom to gently release them from the base and then push them into your prepared hole, pressing the edges of the soil to secure them. Give them a good watering straight after planting them, and ensure they're getting at least four hours of sunshine a day.

Herbs need to be harvested and pruned when they get too tall or 'leggy'; cut them close above the leaf intersections so that they regrow.

SIX SIMPLE HERBS TO GROW

If you're a novice gardener, or have managed to annihilate even the hardiest of house plants, or you have a tendency to neglect windowsill herbs positioned at eye level in the kitchen, I want to arm you with this list of six virtually fail-safe container-grown crops. I've chosen them for their usefulness, versatility and ability to withstand even the blackest of thumbs. An easy-to-grow kitchen garden bursting with flavour is simpler than you think. I dehydrate my herbs every few months and give them to friends as gifts.

Basil

This hardy plant grows best in full sunlight, inside or outside. It loves well-drained but moist soil, and in full swing requires regular pruning to allow for new growth. I use it daily for salads, pesto, pizza toppings and on a slice of supercharged loaf.

Lavender

This is such a fantastic plant to grow as part of your edible garden. Its flowers have so many uses, from tea to baking and even as a natural bathroom fragrance or drawer freshener. Use it on your dining table for an aromatic and visual bonanza. Grow it in a sunny spot in well-drained soil. Prune regularly to keep it under control.

Mint

If you want a super-fast-growing aromatic herb and a fantastic fragrant addition to your edible garden, plant mint. It enjoys a good dose of sun but will also tolerate shade. It's one of my favourite herbs in the garden and a handy plant to have around. When planting, ensure you give it enough space to allow for its rapid growth, and weed out seedlings or it will spread everywhere. I love to make mint tea, but I also use mint in a variety of different dishes, including my strawberry granita, drinks, mint sauce, green salads and Asian stir-fries.

Parsley

A hardy, versatile herb that flourishes in sunny areas and can also do well in shade. The two basic varieties of parsley are flat-leaf (Italian) and curly, and both are easy to grow in pots and in the garden. Plant in spring and water moderately; it grows slower than other herbs but will readily provide plentiful sprigs for you to chop and scatter over a variety of dishes.

Rosemary

Sitting at the top of the list of the easiest herbs to grow is rosemary, especially if it's in a good sunny spot and is watered frequently but left to dry out between waterings. It's happy to live in pots or containers but does grow tall and wide. Its fragrant piny aroma complements winter bakes, soups and casseroles, and it's also lovely sprinkled on pizza.

Thyme

Thyme, a member of the mint family, is an evergreen hardy herb with small but plentiful flowers. It has a piny and peppery taste with bitter, slightly lemony and minty notes. Grow thyme in well-drained soil and plant it in late spring in an area that provides full sun. Thyme grows well indoors too, but ensure it has access to sunlight. Harvest regularly – just pick sprigs off and use them when needed. It gives a delicious boost of flavour to pork, lamb, chicken and fish. I also add it to my oven-roasted sweet potatoes, and to casseroles, stuffing, tomato sauces, slow-cooking, soups and baking.

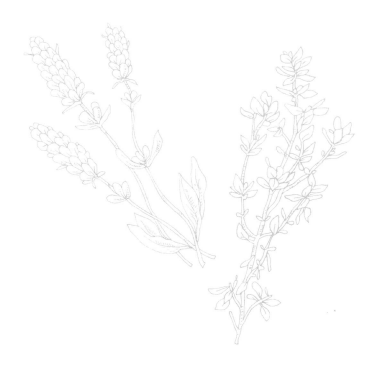

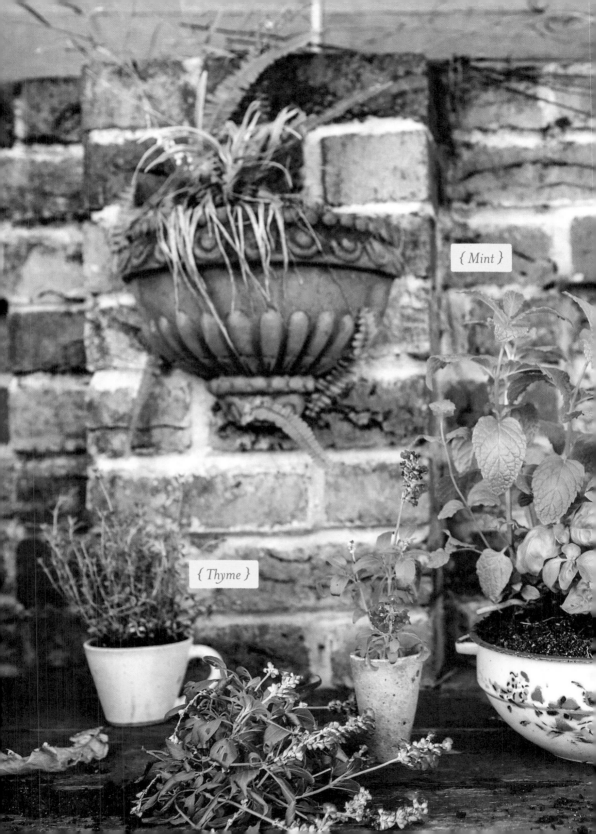

{ Mint }

{ Thyme }

Goat's cheese, tomato and spinach muffins

{ *MAKES 6* }

25 g (1 oz) butter, plus extra for greasing

200 ml (7 fl oz) almond milk

100 g (3½ oz/2¼ cups) baby English spinach leaves, chopped

250 g (9 oz/2½ cups) almond meal

2 teaspoons gluten-free baking powder

1 teaspoon bicarbonate of soda (baking soda)

20 g (¾ oz/¼ cup) nutritional yeast flakes

1 egg, lightly beaten

180 g (6¼ oz/1½ cups) crumbled goat's cheese

175 g (6 oz) roma (plum) tomatoes, halved

1 tablespoon chopped basil leaves

Preheat the oven to 190°C (375°F) and lightly grease a six-hole small muffin tray with butter.

Heat the butter and almond milk in a small saucepan over medium heat. Add the spinach and stir until wilted. Remove from the heat, cool slightly and set aside.

Sift the almond meal, baking powder and bicarbonate of soda into a large bowl. Stir in the yeast flakes, then the egg and the spinach mixture. Crumble in the cheese, then stir gently until just combined.

Divide the tomatoes between the holes in the muffin tray, spoon the muffin mixture over the top and scatter over the basil.

Bake for 20 minutes, or until cooked through, testing with a skewer. Turn out onto a wire rack and enjoy warm.

Sweet potato, broccoli and ham soup

{ *SERVES* 4 }

This soup is so delicious and easy to throw together. It's also great to freeze, for use as a quick midweek work meal. In my eyes, ham is one of the most scrumptious, joyous, flavour-filled foods in the world. But not all hams are created equal. Make sure you find a passionate butcher and invest in quality free-range or organic nitrate-free ham, which will be browner and not so pink (pink ham has been treated with nitrates). The taste is second to none, and you only need small amounts to bring an immense salty ham flavour to your meals.

1 tablespoon olive oil

2 leeks, pale part only, thinly sliced

2 garlic cloves, finely chopped

4 thin nitrate-free ham slices, chopped

500 g (1 lb 2 oz) sweet potato, peeled and chopped

1 turnip, chopped

1 head broccoli, chopped

1 litre (35 fl oz/4 cups) vegetable stock or filtered water

2 teaspoons picked thyme leaves, plus extra sprigs to serve

sea salt and freshly ground black pepper, to taste

80 ml (2½ fl oz/⅓ cup) coconut cream

Heat the olive oil in a large saucepan over medium heat, then cook the leeks, garlic and ham for 5 minutes, stirring frequently. Add the remaining ingredients except the coconut cream, then bring to the boil. Reduce the heat to low and simmer, covered, for 20 minutes, or until the vegetables are cooked.

Transfer half the soup to a blender, allow to cool slightly, then purée until smooth. Return the puréed soup to the pan to heat through.

Ladle into bowls, swirl in the coconut cream and serve garnished with thyme sprigs and a grind of pepper.

SUPERCHARGED TIP
Roasted sweet potato slices make a lovely garnish for this soup, as do edible flowers.

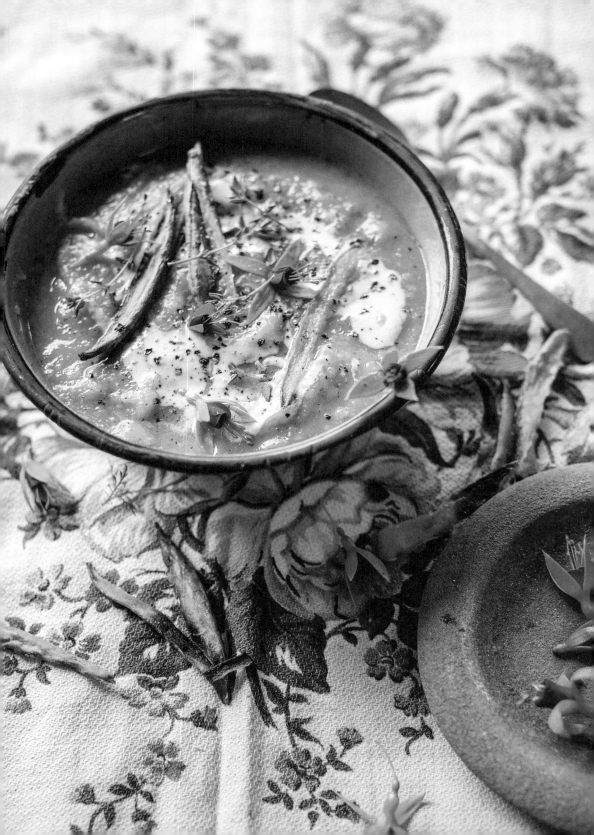

Kale and blood orange salad

{ SERVES 4 AS A SIDE }

Kale has been blitzed into gag-worthy smoothies for far too long. Here, it's redeemed in a tasty salad, paired with bright and zingy blood oranges. This unique crimson-coloured orange develops its distinctive shade when the fruit grows in low overnight temperatures. This brings with it a delightful raspberry-like flavour that adds an unforgettable twist to green salads.

3 blood oranges, 2 peeled and sliced into rounds, 1 juiced

350 g (12 oz/1 small bunch) kale, stems and spines removed

60 ml (2 fl oz/¼ cup) extra virgin olive oil

sea salt and freshly ground black pepper, to taste

2 French shallots, very thinly sliced

1 large carrot, grated (optional)

75 g (2¾ oz/½ cup) pepitas (pumpkin seeds), toasted

15 g (½ oz/¼ cup) coconut flakes, toasted

edible flowers, to serve (optional)

Carefully remove and discard any seeds from the orange slices.

Wash and dry the kale, then massage in half the olive oil to soften.

To make a dressing, combine the orange juice and remaining olive oil in a small bowl, and season with salt and pepper.

Arrange the orange slices and vegetables on a platter, scatter over the pepitas, coconut flakes and edible flowers, if using, and drizzle over the dressing.

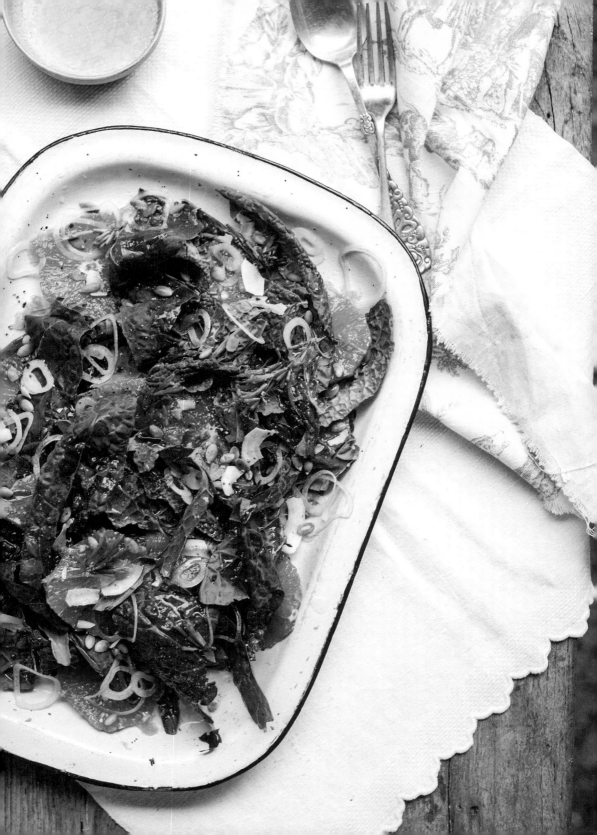

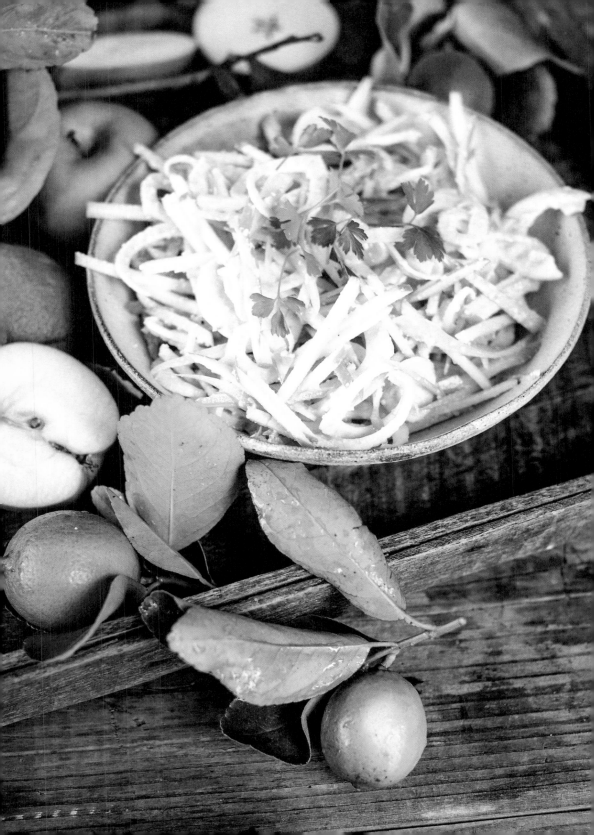

Fennel and apple slaw with mustard dressing

{ SERVES 4 }

3 celery stalks, thinly sliced lengthways

2 small fennel bulbs, cut into matchsticks

1 firm, crisp granny smith apple, cut into matchsticks

50 g (1¾ oz/⅓ cup) sesame seeds, toasted

sea salt and freshly ground black pepper, to taste

coriander (cilantro) leaves, to serve (optional)

Mustard dressing

120 g (4¼ oz/¾ cup) raw cashews, soaked in filtered water for 2 hours

40 g (1½ oz/¼ cup) sesame seeds

1 tablespoon lemon or lime juice

50 ml (1¾ fl oz) tablespoons apple cider vinegar

¼ teaspoon Celtic sea salt

2 tablespoons sugar-free mustard

To make the dressing, blend all the ingredients and a generous splash of filtered water in a food processor until smooth.

Toss the slaw ingredients together in a large bowl, stir through the dressing, top with coriander, if using, and serve.

Farmers' basket with coconut, lime and almond dressing

{ *SERVES* 3-4 }

I find that farmers' market shopping adds an element of wonder and contentment to my life. Apart from the social benefits and getting to meet my food producers face to face, nothing brings me more joy than getting home with a big haul of seasonal produce and making that first meal with the freshest ingredients. This farmers' basket is that recipe. It's one to bless your family with – they'll enjoy the unadulterated innocence of colourful ingredients ripe with the fullest flavour.

2 tomatoes, diced

1 green capsicum (pepper), roasted, then skinned and seeded

1 cucumber, diced

1 zucchini (courgette), diced

1 avocado, peeled and sliced

155 g (5½ oz/1 firmly packed cup) grated carrot

150 g (5½ oz) green beans, steamed

140 g (5 oz/1 cup) diced celery

90 g (3½ oz/2 cups) baby English spinach leaves

coriander (cilantro) leaves and flaked almonds, to serve

Dressing

170 ml (5½ fl oz/²/₃ cup) coconut water

2 tablespoons almond butter

1 tablespoon lime juice

1 teaspoon crushed garlic

1 teaspoon grated fresh ginger

1 teaspoon ground cumin

1 tablespoon wheat-free tamari

sea salt, to taste

To make the dressing, combine all the dressing ingredients in a small bowl and mix with a fork.

Toss all the salad ingredients except the coriander and almonds together and drizzle over the dressing. Scatter over the coriander and almonds to serve.

Microherb and watermelon teacup salad

{ *SERVES* 2 }

120 g (4¼ oz/2 cups) mixed
microherbs, washed and
patted dry

2 slices watermelon, peeled
and diced

½ avocado, peeled and diced

45 g (1½ oz/½ cup) grated
daikon (mooli)

30 g (1 oz/¼ cup) chopped
walnuts

Dressing

1 French shallot, finely diced

1 garlic clove, finely chopped
(optional)

1 tablespoon extra virgin olive
oil

1 tablespoon apple cider
vinegar

1 tablespoon lemon juice

small pinch each of sea salt and
freshly ground black pepper

To make the dressing, combine all the
ingredients in a screw-top jar, then seal and
shake well.

Share the microherbs between large teacups
then top with the remaining ingredients. Pour
over the dressing and serve.

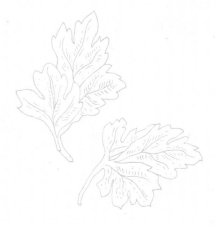

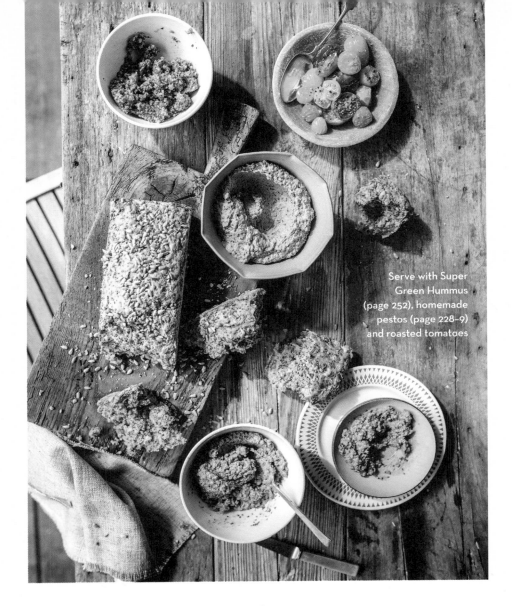

Serve with Super
Green Hummus
(page 252), homemade
pestos (page 228–9)
and roasted tomatoes

Pull-apart green bread

{ *MAKES* 9 x 30 *CM* [3½ x 12 *INCH*] *LOAF* }

This outrageous green beauty has recently become a brand-new staple in my
supercharged kitchen. It's the perfect pull-apart bread to tear and share, and
fantastic for mopping up soup or enjoying with an endless variety of toppings
or leftovers. Packed with greens and fresh herbs, it's also a good sandwich
option, and one that's simple to make. Experiment with your favourite herbs
and seasonings. I enjoy mine topped with hummus and oven-roasted tomatoes.

500 g (1 lb 2 oz) gluten-free self-raising flour (see tip)

¼ teaspoon sea salt

1½ teaspoons gluten-free baking powder

¼ teaspoon bicarbonate of soda (baking soda)

large handful baby English spinach leaves

3 kale leaves, spines removed

handful chives, snipped

75 g (2¾ oz/½ cup) sunflower seeds, plus extra to decorate

2 tablespoons chopped fresh thyme

2 tablespoons chopped fresh oregano

3 eggs, whisked

270 ml (9½ fl oz) coconut milk

1 teaspoon lemon juice

60 g (2¼ oz) unsalted butter, melted

1 tablespoon apple cider vinegar

Preheat the oven to 175°C (345°F) and line a 9 × 30 cm (3½ × 12 inch) loaf (bar) tin with baking paper.

In a large bowl, combine the flour, salt, baking powder and bicarbonate of soda.

Whiz the spinach and kale in a food processor (or chop them finely) and add to the bowl, along with all of the remaining ingredients. Mix thoroughly.

Spoon the mixture into the prepared tin and level the surface with the back of a spoon dipped in cold water.

Bake on the middle shelf of the oven for about 45 minutes, until a skewer inserted in the centre comes out clean. Halfway through cooking, scatter the extra sunflower seeds on top – they'll go all nice and crunchy.

Turn out onto a wire rack to cool, then enjoy. The bread will keep for up to 1 week in an airtight container in the fridge, or can be frozen for up to 1 month.

SUPERCHARGED TIP

Make your own self-raising gluten-free flour by mixing equal quantities (or your preferred proportions) of almond meal, brown rice flour and tapioca flour. Add 1 teaspoon baking powder and ¼ teaspoon bicarbonate of soda (baking soda) for every 2½ cups of flour.

If making your own flour, you won't need the baking powder or bicarbonate of soda in the main ingredients list.

Pasta the pesto please

Triple the pleasure with pesto three ways. Serve on eggs, crackers or flatbread, add to pasta or pizza, or serve as an accompaniment to chicken or fish dishes. Pestos are a must with pasta, and for this reason I'm sure to include them in my weekly menu plan. I like to prepare batches of different pestos each week. These pestos will keep in a sealed container in the fridge for up to 1 week, and can be refreshed with an extra splash of extra virgin olive oil.

Cashew and basil pesto

{ *MAKES ABOUT 250 G [9 OZ/1 CUP]* }

155 g (5½ oz/1 cup) raw cashews, soaked in filtered water for 2 hours

2 garlic cloves, peeled

2 large handfuls basil leaves

80 ml (2½ fl oz/⅓ cup) extra virgin olive oil

1 teaspoon grated lemon zest

1 tablespoon lemon juice

2 tablespoons nutritional yeast flakes

small pinch of sea salt

Whiz the cashews in a food processor until chunky. Add the garlic and pulse, then add the basil and whiz again. With the motor running, slowly drizzle in the olive oil until the mixture has the desired consistency, then add the lemon zest and juice, yeast flakes and salt.

Spinach and hazelnut pesto

{ *MAKES ABOUT* 375 *G* [13 *OZ* / 1½ *CUPS*] }

This pesto takes a unique angle with the earthy flavours of roasted hazelnuts combined with glowing green spinach.

75 g (2³/₄ oz/¹/₂ cup) roasted hazelnuts

90 g (3¹/₄ oz/2 cups) baby English spinach leaves

large handful basil leaves

20 g (³/₄ oz/¹/₄ cup) nutritional yeast flakes

grated zest of ¹/₂ lemon

2 tablespoons lemon juice

1 garlic clove, chopped

sea salt and freshly ground black pepper, to taste

90 ml (3 fl oz) olive oil

Whiz the hazelnuts in a food processor until chunky. Add the remaining ingredients except the olive oil and pulse, then slowly drizzle in the oil until the mixture has the desired consistency. Refrigerate for a few hours for the flavours to develop.

Rocket and macadamia pesto

{ *MAKES ABOUT* 375 *G* [13 *OZ* / 1½ *CUPS*] }

115 g (4 oz/³/₄ cup) roasted salted macadamia nuts

2 garlic cloves, peeled

130 g (4¹/₂ oz) rocket (arugula)

60 ml (2 fl oz/¹/₄ cup) olive oil

1 teaspoon grated lemon zest

2 tablespoons lemon juice

2 tablespoons nutritional yeast flakes

small pinch of sea salt

Whiz the macadamia nuts and garlic in a food processor until coarsely chopped. Add the rocket and pulse until finely chopped but not puréed. With the motor running, slowly drizzle in the olive oil until the mixture has the desired consistency, then add the lemon zest and juice, yeast flakes and salt.

Asparagus, mushroom and salmon frittata

{ *SERVES* 4 }

8 eggs

125 ml (4 fl oz/½ cup) almond milk

½ teaspoon sea salt

2 tablespoons nutritional yeast flakes (optional)

200 g (7 oz) cooked salmon, flaked

90 g (3¼ oz) mushrooms, sautéed

350 g (12 oz/2 bunches) asparagus, woody ends trimmed, blanched

sea salt and freshly ground black pepper, to taste

chives, finely chopped, to serve (optional)

Preheat the oven to 180°C (350°F) and grease a 22 cm (8½ inch) pie dish or 15 × 25 cm (6 × 10 inch) baking tin.

Whisk the eggs in a large bowl, then whisk in the almond milk, salt and yeast flakes, if using. Spread the salmon in the prepared pie dish and pour the egg mixture over. Arrange the mushrooms and asparagus on top.

Bake for 25-30 minutes, or until the frittata is set in the middle and the top is puffy and slightly browned.

Serve hot or cold, seasoned with salt and pepper, and topped with chives, if using.

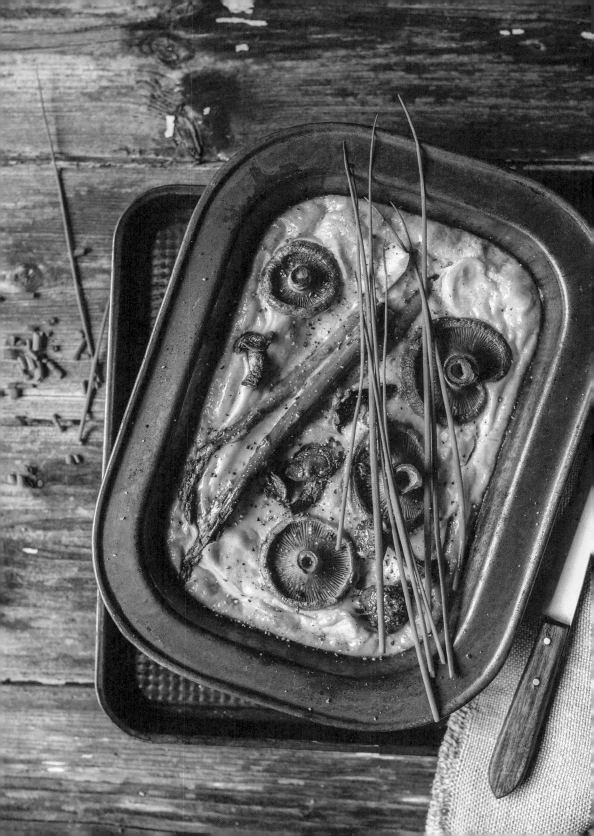

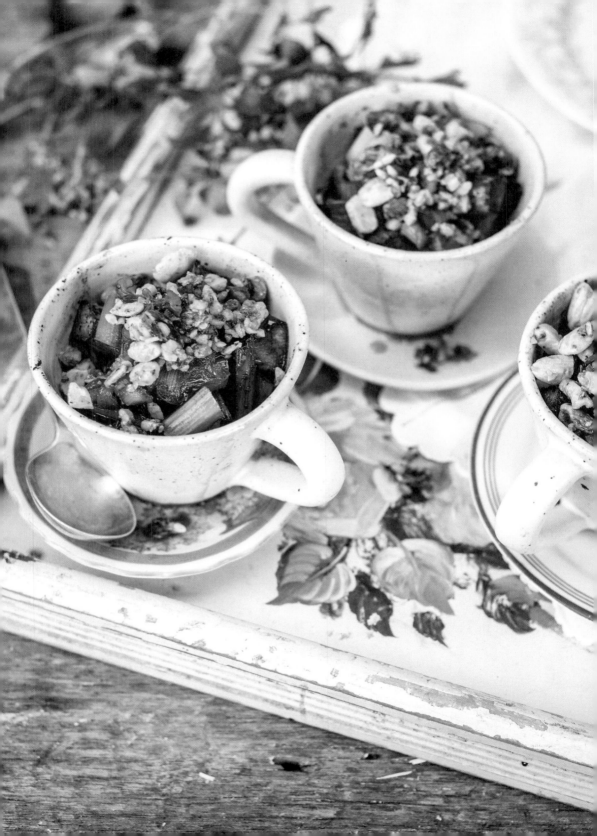

Rhubarb crumble pies

{ *SERVES* 4 }

I can't go past a crumble when I'm in need of a quick dessert for friends or family. I love how versatile they are, and I often use seasonal fruits and also chop and change my crumble ingredients depending on which dry whole foods I have in my pantry. This recipe celebrates the glory of rhubarb, which peaks in autumn and winter.

600 g (1 lb 5 oz/1 bunch) rhubarb, trimmed and cut into 5–7.5 cm (2–3 inch) lengths

75 g (2¾ oz/½ cup) coconut sugar

grated zest and juice of 1 orange

1 × 2.5 cm (1 inch) piece fresh ginger, grated

1 teaspoon vanilla powder

60 ml (2 fl oz/¼ cup) filtered water

½ teaspoon freshly grated nutmeg

½ teaspoon ground cinnamon

185 g (6½ oz/1½ cups) walnuts, 240 g (8½ oz/1½ cups) almonds or 210 g (7½ oz/ 1½ cups) mixed nuts

60 g (2¼ oz) butter, diced

pinch of sea salt

chilled coconut cream or Coconut 'Yoghurt' (page 195), to serve (optional)

edible flowers, to serve (optional)

Preheat the oven to 175°C (345°F). Grease four individual pie dishes or ovenproof teacups.

Put the rhubarb in a large saucepan with 50 g (1¾ oz/⅓ cup) of the coconut sugar, and the orange zest and juice, ginger, vanilla powder and water. Bring to the boil over medium heat, then reduce the heat to low and simmer gently for about 10 minutes, until the rhubarb is soft but still holding its shape.

Add the nutmeg, cinnamon and remaining coconut sugar. Divide the rhubarb between the prepared dishes or cups.

Finely chop the nuts in a food processor, if using. Add the butter and salt, and mix until crumbly. Scatter the mixture over the rhubarb. Bake for 15–20 minutes, until crispy on top.

Serve topped with edible flowers and chilled coconut cream or coconut 'yoghurt' on the side, if using.

Fruit roll-ups

Fruit roll-ups are super easy to make, and you can use a multitude of fruit combinations to fit in with the seasons. Frozen fruit works well too.

Strawberry and chia roll-up

{ *MAKES ABOUT* 12 }

500 g (1 lb 2 oz/3⅓ cups) strawberries, hulled and halved

2 tablespoons chia seeds

2 tablespoons rice malt syrup, or stevia powder to taste

OTHER GREAT COMBINATIONS

RASPBERRY + MANGO

APPLE + SWEET POTATO

PEACH + BANANA

STRAWBERRY + BASIL

APPLE + GINGER

RASPBERRY + VANILLA

APRICOT + CINNAMON + TURMERIC

Preheat the oven to 65°C (145°F) or its lowest temperature and line two baking trays with baking paper.

Combine all the ingredients in a food processor and pulse for about 30 seconds, until puréed. Pour onto the baking trays and spread out evenly with a spatula.

Dry in the oven for at least 3 hours, until the mixture is no longer sticky and the consistency is leathery but not crisp (see tip).

Cool to room temperature, then either slowly peel the fruit off the baking paper or use a sharp knife or a pair of scissors to cut into portions with the paper still on to stop them sticking. Store in an airtight container in the fridge for 3–4 days. When ready to use, roll up portions and secure with string.

SUPERCHARGED TIP

To test whether your fruit roll-up is ready, pick at a corner and start to peel it slowly off the paper. If it pulls apart or seems sticky or damp, it needs to go back in the oven. To make the other flavour combinations, replace the strawberries with the same volume of the suggested ingredients, and combine with the chia seeds and rice malt syrup in the same way.

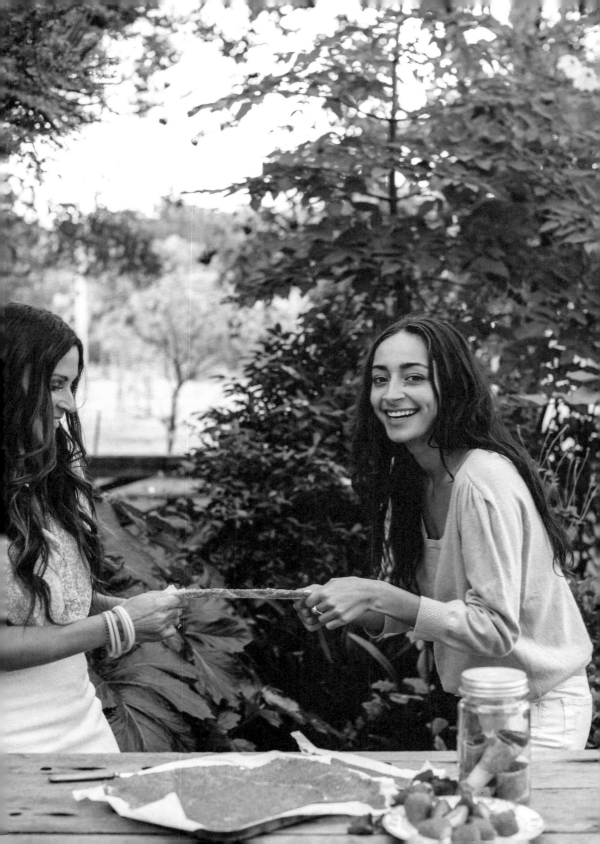

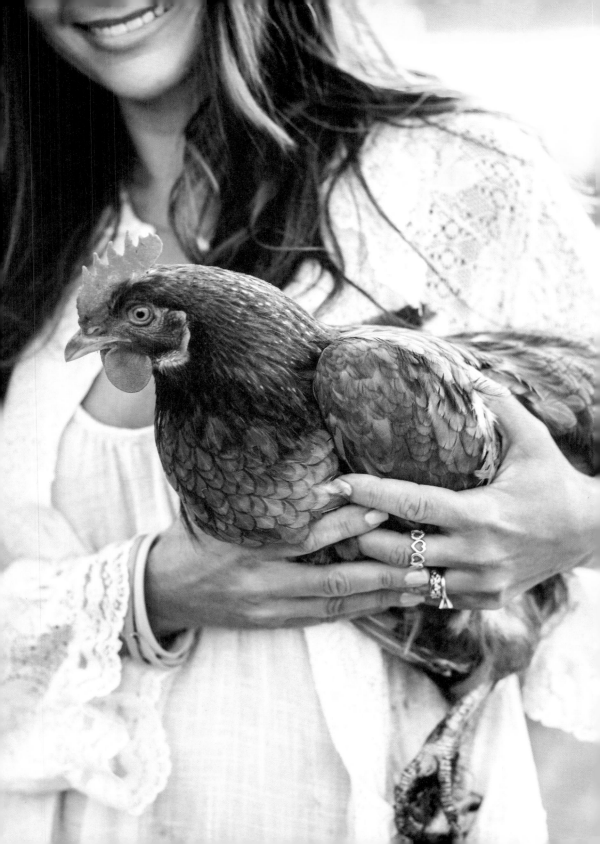

Consuming with purpose

Sadly, our food systems are in trouble. With the rise of the supermarket, economic principles better suited to manufacturing and mass production of non-perishable goods have been applied to food in the name of fat profit margins for multinational corporations.

The people who are benefiting are far removed from the damaging realities of this process for farmers and the environment. Food has been transformed from something we were once in tune with and connected to – something we loved and respected – into a commodity. This reversal has generated lower food prices as a result of the economies of scale, but our hyper-efficient and growth-dependent food system is flooding our supermarket shelves and our food culture with unnecessary fad foods and foods of poor nutritional value and quality. We're eating cheap ingredients derived from wheat and soya beans in quantities and forms that were never seen in traditional cultures, where people ate a time-honoured diet and prepared their foods with love and care.

The 'success' of our modern food system is ironically built on the necessity for farmers to enter a vicious cycle of hardship. High-volume and low-cost production by large food companies locks farmers into a pattern of increasing demand for higher yields at lower costs in order to allow competitive prices. The farmer will invest in technology and machinery to help achieve this growing demand. The technology is expensive. The farmer accumulates debt, and all the farmers around will match this investment to produce more of their own crops, with the aim of spreading the costs over greater yield. The mass effect of farmers doing this increases the total supply of one crop. As supply rises faster than demand, prices fall, and farmers are trapped into investing in still more technology, creating more debt for themselves without a fair income flowing in.

Take food to heart. It's time to look at food and shopping as a purposeful act.

Where you shop matters. Mass production methods and practices may mean you get food at a cheap price, but behind the scenes they're having dire consequences for farmers, the land and soil quality, and the health of our nations. With this in mind, you can understand the beauty and fulfilment that can come from being intentional about your food purchases.

INVEST IN YOUR WORLD

Having good intentions means you can pave a new way, and have a purposeful and direct effect by breaking some of the harmful practices of our food systems. You can also help to ensure the wellbeing and protection of farmers, an increase in fair pricing, and increased access to local fresh food free from harmful chemicals. This will have a ripple effect of improving health and access to fair food in your local community.

Where you choose to spend your money is a direct and daily vote for the kind of world you want to live in. Living a supercharged life is, in essence, living from the heart and through your value system and food culture. How wonderful that the simple everyday act of choosing food can be full of such purpose and significance! When you live a life with this kind of intent, the result is a heart filled with passion and joy, and a happier and healthier, more connected community.

See your food budget as an investment in your world.

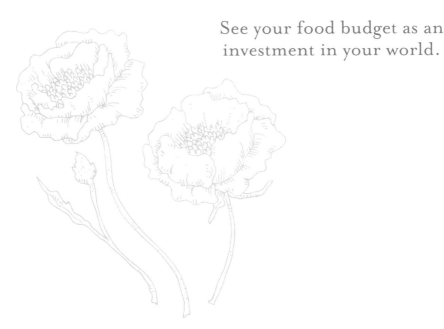

Enriching your community

Food and community go hand in hand. Sit a bunch of strangers around a bare table and I can guarantee a level of awkwardness. But spread food in front of them and the atmosphere will shift to one of warmth, conversation and connection. The focus shifts away from the individual towards the food and the shared experience of enjoyment.

Not only does eating draw people together, but even the small act of where you shop can bring about greater connections to people in your local area – to new friends and like-minded people, not to mention local farmers and food producers from whom you can source very affordable fresh food.

According to psychologist Abraham Maslow, when all our basic needs in life are met (remember those seven keystones of life?) we come to a point where we can reach our full potential (a process Maslow called self-actualisation), and enter a realm of self-discovery and self-exploration. Your purposeful food journey can lead you down a path, as it has done for me, that will enable you to discover more and more about your own potential to become an agent for change – for yourself and those around you. That might be through blogging, starting a business or a social enterprise that builds meaningful connections between food and community, or just cooking great food for those around you. The possibilities are endless.

By reaching a level of self-actualisation, you can create a Mexican wave that spills over into inspiring other people. This has the power to generate more empathy within your community, and through your example you may even be able to motivate a shift in that community towards kinder and more thoughtful food choices, without you having to be evangelical in your approach. On the next few pages are some ideas to help you achieve this.

Start with your inner circle

Supercharging the lives of those around you and attempting to be a food-change agent can seem like a big task, but the best way to create change in a community is to work from yourself outwards. The first thing you can do is learn self-leadership. This will have an impact on your family or your close inner circle of influence.

It could involve starting to cook from scratch for your family or household, having a meal-planning day once a week, doing research on local food producers, or joining a food co-op and gathering your food from farmers' markets or online organic delivery services instead of supermarkets.

Potluck gatherings are also a great way to create community and expose your friends to a range of foods they may never have tried before. They're also lots of fun, and when everyone feels like they've contributed to the feast, there tends to be a greater appreciation for the food and the cooking of others. Next time you're having a celebration or gathering of friends, ask everyone to bring their own plate of food. It will save you lots of time and energy. For some picnic recipes and simple picnic-scape ideas, turn to pages 245–65 and 337.

Over time, these small steps will have an ever greater impact on your own and your family's wellbeing, which other people will notice and find inspirational. They will start asking you questions and the chain reaction will begin.

Get out into the community

You can also influence your community through partnering and supporting local groups and businesses that stand for similar values to your own.

You may have local political food fairness groups that provide education and direct opportunities for you to impact local food systems. You might like to join a cooking class on how to prepare real food, or become a member and volunteer at your local food co-op or community garden. My kitchen garden, for example, has attracted many visitors, who can come and take the herbs they need. It also encourages them to cook, too, spreading the supercharged message further.

These kinds of connections will gradually enhance your knowledge of real food and where to find it, and will open up opportunities for you to contribute further to great food-related causes in your area. You'll also develop meaningful relationships with people that will propel your journey of self-actualisation forward.

Express yourself further

When your tide of influence has extended out into your community, you may come to a point in your journey where you've learnt so much that you feel the desire to express it and share it with others. This is why I started blogging. My motive was simply to share all the things I'd learnt, and the momentum propelled me from there. I'm incredibly thankful that this has allowed me to find alignment between my passion and what I do for a living, and created a gravitational pull that has brought me so many new friends and an inspiring community.

I liken living a supercharged life to a radio wave that embodies your authentic self, radiating outwards without hype or evangelicalism, that gently rubs off on others. This, alongside understanding and recognising others' viewpoints, even when they oppose your own, can be a catalyst for finding common ground and for collaboration.

CREATING A RADIO WAVE

The metamodern approach doesn't pave over our differences in food culture or choices, but simply emphasises areas of overlap between contesting opinions, which can act as a precedent for collective action. The radio wave looks like this:

- You enthuse your immediate family and friends.
- This enthusiasm permeates into the community.
- It moves from community to country.
- It spreads from country to the world.

Your wave may look different from mine. You may want to begin your own social enterprise, an organic food business, or a local club or group that helps others on their food journey. You might want to write for a local newspaper, run meal-planning workshops, develop an app or a guide for your city that connects people to local food producers, or study health coaching or nutrition. The world really is your oyster.

At this point you've moved from self-leadership to family leadership, then to influencing your friends and your community, extending out into your city, nation and even the world. Who knows where it could take you?

You just need to keep it simple and start from within. But to do this you'll need to embody a sense of wild abandonment and freedom when it comes to the food you choose to eat. This will allow you to recognise and support the views of others. Think of empathy and equality as the opposing force to passive-aggressive tolerance of others and their opinions. We don't get to choose whether someone else's viewpoint matters, it just does, and we need a dynamic dialogue between opposing ideas and mindsets to move forward.

Before you can do this, turn to the next section, to learn how to liberate and supercharge your attitudes surrounding food, and connect food to the seven keystones of life. You'll start by learning how to depollute your mind of unhelpful thinking about food. It's time to join the dots and connect.

But first, you're ready to gather and feast, here's a bunch of recipes for delightful things to take along to gatherings, potlucks and picnics.

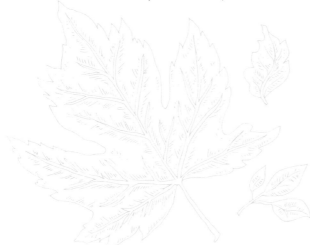

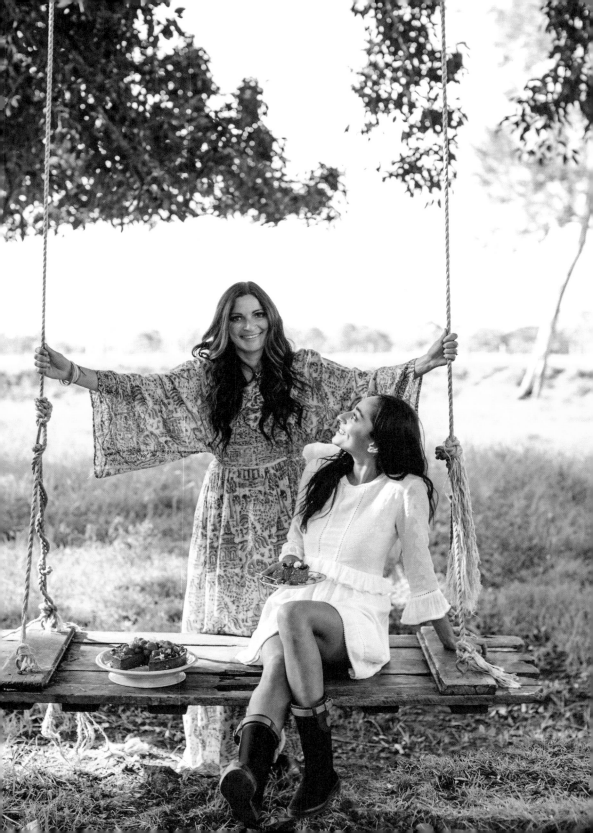

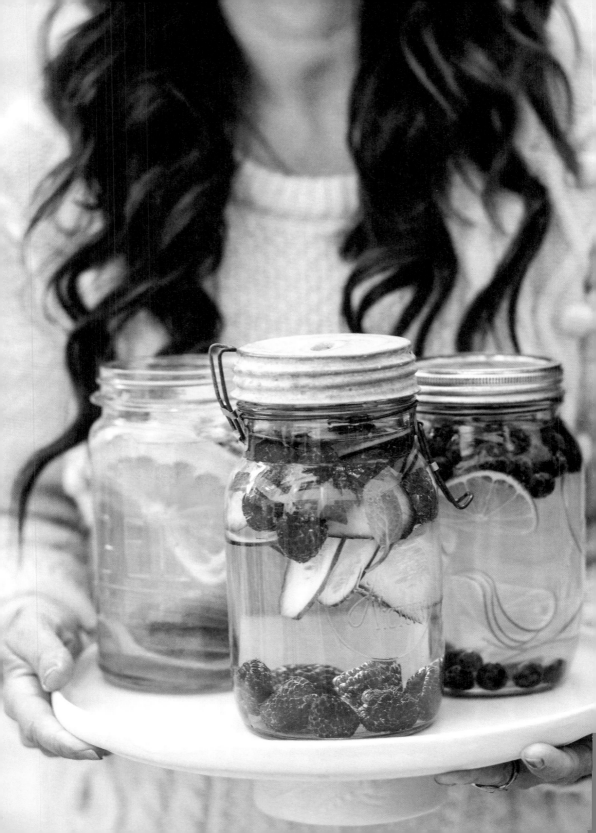

How to create supercharged water jars

These jars just scream summer holidays! It's time to leave vitamin waters, reconstituted fruit juices and sports drinks back where they belong – on the supermarket shelves. Really, it's super easy to create your own jars of infused water and stay refreshed through the warm summer months. Why not take full advantage of summer fruits and herbs to enliven your daily water intake and ensure continuous hydration?

They're wonderful for entertaining, too, and look gorgeous on a table or sideboard. Flip over to the tablescape section (page 315) for some ideas on how to create beautiful settings.

For your infused waters, you'll need a screw-top glass jar and perhaps a paper straw. Look for fresh ingredients, and avoid overripe or heavily bruised fruit and veg. There are four steps to creating a delicious infused water (although depending on your combo only two or three might apply), and the secret is to mix and match and tweak to suit your personal preferences.

1   Start building your jar with a base of seasonal fruit, remembering to give all your ingredients a good rinse beforehand. You can include peeled and sliced lemon, lime, grapefruit, orange, mandarin, all types of berries, mango and other tropical fruits, kiwi fruit, pomegranate or other favourite fruits, such as apple, grapes, peach, nectarine or pear. Removing the peel from citrus reduces bitterness, while using thin slices enables a faster infusion.

2   Next, tumble some vegetables into your jar and push them down with a wooden spoon to release their flavours. I like to use sliced or halved cucumber and fennel, and sliced carrots or celery stalks.

3   Next choose your herbs. Some that work well are rosemary, basil, mint, thyme, sage and coriander (cilantro). Take them in your hand and squeeze them gently to bruise them, releasing their natural aroma and oils. You can also add whole spices to the mix, such as cinnamon sticks, cardamom pods, nutmeg, a vanilla bean, cloves and fresh ginger slices. Also fun are edible blossoms, such as rose, lavender, citrus flowers, hibiscus, pansies and violets, but make sure they're food-grade and pesticide-free. >

4 Last, pour in filtered water or, if you prefer, sparkling mineral water on top and let it sit for a few hours until infused. Or you could use coconut water instead. Some flavours take longer to infuse than others. Generally, citrus is fairly quick but some herbs need longer, and berries can take a while to colour the water. You can also leave them in the fridge overnight to infuse further.

Try the delicious combinations below or the two recipes opposite.

BLUEBERRY + LEMON + MINT

ORANGE + CARDAMOM + CINNAMON + CLOVE + ALLSPICE

STRAWBERRY + BASIL + VANILLA

LEMON + STRAWBERRY + BASIL

GRAPEFRUIT + ROSEMARY

PEAR + FENNEL

LEMON + BASIL

STRAWBERRY + LIME + BASIL

RASPBERRY + THYME + ROSE PETALS

LEMON + LIME + ORANGE + MINT

LEMON + GINGER

PINEAPPLE + CUCUMBER + MINT

MANDARIN + PEAR + MINT OR CORIANDER (CILANTRO)

LEMON + ORANGE + GINGER

BLOOD ORANGE + BASIL + GINGER

LIME + CUCUMBER + MINT

GRAPEFRUIT + CUCUMBER + SAGE

WATERMELON + CUCUMBER + MINT

APPLE + LEMON + CARROT + GINGER

POMEGRANATE + CARROT + SAGE

WATERMELON + BASIL

BANANA + BLUEBERRY + BASIL

BLACKBERRY + RASPBERRY + STRAWBERRY + MINT

STRAWBERRY + GRAPEFRUIT + SAGE

APPLE + BLUEBERRY + MINT

Lemon, strawberry and basil water jar

{ *SERVES* 1 }

150 g (5½ oz/1 cup)
   strawberries, hulled and
   halved

squeeze of lemon juice

handful basil leaves

filtered water or sparkling
   mineral water

Place the strawberries in a jar and add the lemon juice. Scrunch the basil leaves in your hands to release their oils and flavour, and gently mix in with a wooden spoon. Fill the jar with water, then seal and leave to infuse.

Apple, raspberry and rosemary water jar

{ *SERVES* 1 }

1 apple, sliced

handful raspberries

several rosemary sprigs

filtered water or sparkling
   mineral water

Place the apple and raspberries in the jar. Bruise the rosemary in your hands and gently mix into the fruit with a wooden spoon. Fill the jar with water, then seal and leave to infuse overnight. Drink the following day.

Sweet lime and ginger cooler

{ *SERVES* 2 }

Perfect for balmy summer evenings, house parties and family gatherings, this striking beverage will really wow your guests as a refreshing and sweet mocktail. The mix of zingy lime and ginger with an innovative cardamom twist will be a real standout, and encourage some curious foodie conversation. Limes assist dutifully with rehydration in the summer months. Make the combo fizzy by using sparkling water with or in place of the coconut water, and take it with you to a party or barbecue.

2 lime cheeks

1 × 2.5 cm (1 inch) piece fresh ginger, sliced

pinch of ground cardamom

500 ml (17 fl oz/2 cups) coconut water

juice of ½ lime

½ teaspoon rice malt syrup, or 6 drops liquid stevia or ⅛ teaspoon stevia powder

crushed ice, to serve

Mix all the ingredients, except the ice, in a jug, and refrigerate for 30 minutes to infuse. Serve chilled over crushed ice.

Note: For a photo of this drink, see page 336–37.

Sesame and cranberry tahini slice

{ *MAKES* 8 }

This scrumptious bake exceeds all expectations of a healthy slice. It's full of interesting flavours, such as sesame and coconut – and cranberries for a sour-sweet burst. I love to make a snack like this once every couple of weeks and freeze it so I have instant access to an interesting sweet treat when friends come over for a cuppa. Life's too short not to bless yourself with sweetness!

290 g (10¼ oz/2 cups) sesame seeds

145 g (5 oz/1 cup) dried cranberries

35 g (1¼ oz/½ cup) shredded coconut

50 g (1¾ oz/½ cup) flaxseed meal

165 g (5¾ oz) tahini

120 g (4¼ oz/⅓ cup) rice malt syrup

60 ml (2 fl oz/¼ cup) coconut oil

1 tablespoon coconut cream

1 teaspoon alcohol-free vanilla extract

¾ teaspoon sea salt

Preheat the oven to 175°C (345°F). Grease a 20 cm (8 inch) square cake tin and line it with baking paper.

Combine the sesame seeds, cranberries, coconut and flaxseed meal in a large bowl and stir well. Add the remaining ingredients and stir to combine.

Turn the mixture out into the prepared tin, then press down firmly using wet hands. Bake for 15–20 minutes.

Cool in the tin then cut into eight bars. Store in an airtight container in the fridge for up to 1 week, or in the freezer for up to 6 months.

Fennel and poppy seed crackers

{ *MAKES* 15–30 }

135 g (4³/₄ oz/1¹/₃ cups) almond meal

80 g (2³/₄ oz/¹/₂ cup) poppy seeds

1 tablespoon fennel seeds

1 teaspoon grated lemon zest

¹/₂ teaspoon sea salt

1 egg

1¹/₂ tablespoons extra virgin olive oil

Preheat the oven to 175°C (345°F) and grease a baking tray.

Combine the almond meal, poppy seeds, fennel seeds, lemon zest and salt in a bowl.

Whisk the egg in a small bowl, then slowly add the olive oil in a thin stream while still whisking. Pour the egg mixture into the dry ingredients and mix to form a firm dough. If it is too dry to roll out, mix in a little filtered water.

Roll the dough out on a sheet of baking paper to a thin rectangle about 35 × 25 cm (14 × 10 inches). Place the prepared baking tray face down over the top, then invert the two together so the dough is in the middle and the paper on top. Peel off the baking paper and cut the dough into squares using a sharp knife.

Bake for 12–15 minutes, until crisp. Allow to cool completely before serving.

Store in an airtight container for 3–4 days.

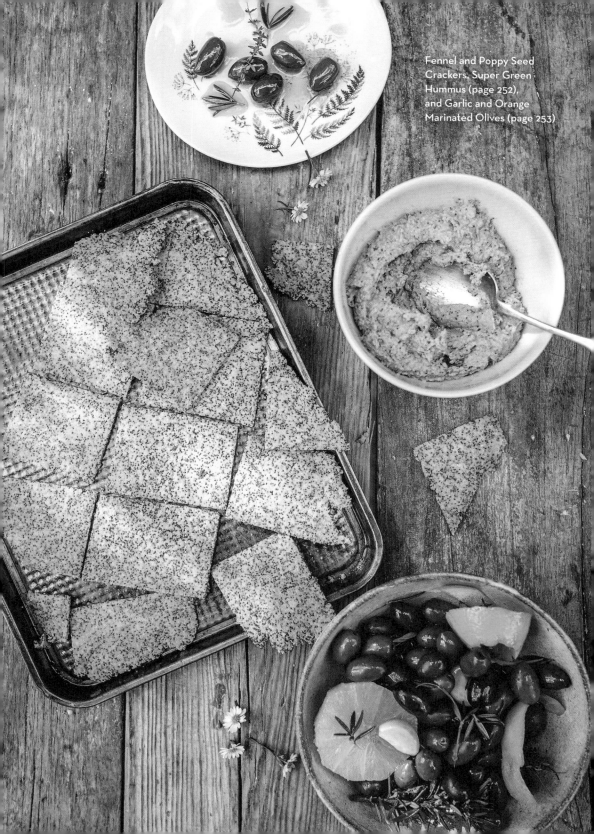

Fennel and Poppy Seed
Crackers, Super Green
Hummus (page 252),
and Garlic and Orange
Marinated Olives (page 253)

Super green hummus

{ *MAKES ABOUT* 440 G [15½ OZ / 2 CUPS] }

Dips are a great way to lift the enjoyment of cheap seasonal vegies and avoid food waste. If you have a few interesting dips on hand, you can jazz up vegies languishing in your crisper by cutting them into crudités and dipping away. I love to make a platter of crudités to serve with this wholesome green hummus as a welcoming and colourful spread for friends. It's a super-speedy hospitality winner.

65 g (2¼ oz/¼ cup) tahini

grated zest and juice of 1 lemon

25 g (1 oz/½ cup) baby English spinach leaves

small handful basil leaves, plus extra, chopped, to serve

small handful rocket (arugula)

1 large garlic clove, roughly chopped

2 tablespoons olive oil, plus extra to serve

½ teaspoon sea salt, plus extra to taste

400 g (14 oz) tinned chickpeas, rinsed and drained

filtered water, as needed

In the bowl of a food processor, combine the tahini, lemon zest and juice, spinach, basil, rocket, garlic, olive oil and salt. Process until the greens are broken down. Add the chickpeas and process until smooth and creamy. Add filtered water if too thick.

Adjust the seasoning before serving drizzled with extra olive oil and with extra basil scattered over. Store in an airtight container in the fridge for up to 1 week.

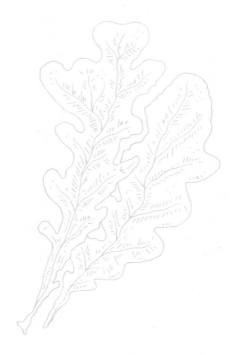

Garlic and orange marinated olives

{ *MAKES 500 G [1 LB 2 OZ]* }

These marinated olives are a super way to turn a regular olive into something you might find in a swanky city bar, all with minimal effort and a few everyday ingredients. Mix these up for your next family gathering – and be prepared to share the recipe, because it will be a talking point!

500 g (1 lb 2 oz) drained kalamata olives

4 rosemary sprigs

4 thyme sprigs

4 garlic cloves, peeled and halved

peel of 1 orange, no pith, cut into wide strips

flesh of ½ orange, roughly chopped

extra virgin olive oil, to cover

Combine all the ingredients except the olive oil in a medium bowl, then transfer to a screw-top preserving jar. Pour in enough olive oil to cover and seal tightly.

Marinate in the fridge for at least 1 hour before enjoying. They'll keep in the fridge for 1 week.

Sesame flat bread

{ MAKES 2 }

100 g (3½ oz/1 cup) almond
meal

75 g (2¾ oz/½ cup) sesame
seeds

¼ teaspoon sea salt

¼ teaspoon gluten-free baking
powder

1 tablespoon extra virgin olive
oil

1 egg, whisked

1 tablespoon apple cider
vinegar

Preheat the oven to 175°C (345°F).

Combine the almond meal, sesame seeds, salt and baking powder in a large bowl. Add the olive oil and, using your fingertips, rub it into the mixture to form a crumble. Add the egg and vinegar, and stir to combine.

Using your hands, take the mixture out of the bowl, transfer to a clean work surface and knead for a few minutes until it forms a smooth dough. It will feel quite sticky at first, but will smooth out as you mix. Divide in half and leave to sit on the work surface for 5–10 minutes.

Cut four 20 cm (8 inch) squares of baking paper and lay one piece on the work surface. Sit one piece of the dough on the baking paper and lay another piece of baking paper on top. Using a rolling pin, roll the dough out into a circle about 15 cm (6 inches) in diameter and about 1 cm (½ inch) thick. Repeat with the other ball of dough and the remaining sheets of baking paper.

Gently peel the top layer of baking paper off one piece of dough, then lift using the bottom sheet of baking paper onto a baking tray. Repeat with the other round of dough and a second tray or bake the two separately, re-using the one tray. Bake for 12 minutes, or until golden.

Remove from the oven, turn onto a wire rack and peel off the baking paper – it should come away quite easily. Cool until crunchy.

This bread will keep in the fridge for 1 week and the freezer for 2 months.

Turmeric sesame crackers

{ MAKES ABOUT 35 }

125 g (4½ oz/1¼ cups) almond
meal

½ teaspoon sea salt

75 g (2¾ oz/½ cup) sesame
seeds

1 teaspoon ground turmeric

1 teaspoon grated lemon zest

1 egg

1½ tablespoons extra virgin
olive oil

Preheat the oven to 175°C (345°F) and grease
a baking tray.

Combine the almond meal, salt, sesame seeds,
turmeric and lemon zest in a large bowl.

In a small bowl, whisk the egg, then slowly add
the olive oil in a thin stream while still whisking.
Pour the egg mixture into the dry ingredients
and mix to form a firm dough. If it is too dry to
roll out, mix in a little filtered water.

Roll the dough out on a sheet of baking paper
to a thin rectangle about 25 × 35 cm (10 ×
14 inches). Place the prepared baking tray
face down over the top then invert the two
together so the dough is in the middle and the
paper on top. Peel off the baking paper and
cut the dough into 5 cm (2 inch) squares using
a sharp knife.

Bake for 12–15 minutes, until crisp. Allow to
cool completely before using.

Keep in an airtight container for 3–4 days.

Lemony goat's cheese dip

{ MAKES ABOUT 375 G [13 OZ] }

220 g (7³/₄ oz/1 cup) hummus or Super Green Hummus (page 252)

150 g (5¹/₂ oz) goat's cheese

2 tablespoons olive oil

1 teaspoon lemon zest

1 tablespoon lemon juice

sea salt and freshly ground black pepper, to taste

pita chips, Omega Cheese Crackers (below) or 'Cheesy' Tomato and Basil Braids (page 279), to serve

Mix all the ingredients in a food processor. Serve with pita chips, omega cheese crackers or 'cheesy' tomato and basil braids.

Omega cheese crackers

{ MAKES ABOUT 24 }

Home-made crackers are a great way to save money, save the earth by reducing package waste, and just make dip dunking and snacking so much more gratifying. These crispy flaxseed meal crackers are a weekly bake in my household, and the addition of nutritional yeast flakes gives the tastiest cheesy flavour. Great for entertaining, afternoon snacking and kids' lunchboxes.

200 g (7 oz/2 cups) flaxseed meal

185–250 ml (6–9 fl oz/³/₄–1 cup) filtered water

2 tablespoons coconut aminos

1 tablespoon nutritional yeast flakes (optional)

¹/₈ teaspoon sea salt

Preheat the oven to 180°C (350°F) and line a baking tray with baking paper.

In a medium bowl, combine all the ingredients and mix until they form a smooth dough.

Spread the dough to about 3 mm (¹/₈ inch) thick on the prepared baking tray. Score into squares or diamonds so the crackers can be broken apart easily when baked.

Bake for 20–30 minutes, until crispy.

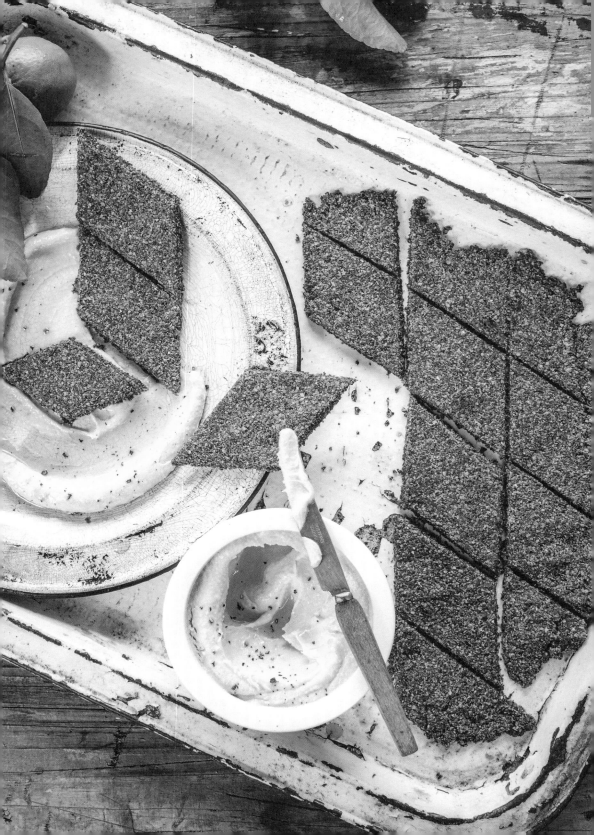

Tri-colour sundried tomatoes

{ MAKES ABOUT 400 G [14 OZ] }

about 750 g (1 lb 10 oz) ripe but firm heirloom red, green and yellow truss tomatoes, or whatever varieties are available

olive oil

sea salt

1 tablespoon chopped or dried basil

Preheat the oven to 75°C (165°F) (see tip).

Cut the tomatoes into uniformly thick slices and place in a bowl. Drizzle with olive oil, sprinkle with salt and basil, and toss gently.

Spread out the tomatoes in a roasting tin and bake for about 3 hours, keeping the door open a crack to allow moisture to escape. After 3 hours, turn the tomatoes over and press flat with a spatula. Return to the oven and continue to dry for at least another hour, until leathery but still pliable.

SUPERCHARGED TIP

You can also use a dehydrator for this recipe. Dehydrate for at least 8 hours.

Sheep's yoghurt dip with pomegranate

{ *MAKES ABOUT 520 G [1 LB 2½ OZ / 2 CUPS]* }

Sheep's milk yoghurt is a beautiful item to have on hand as the basis for a quick dressing or dip. It has a mild, clean flavour that can act as a pure foundation for a range of ingredients. Here, it's bejewelled with bright-pink hits of pomegranate and will bring you so much pleasure as you dunk in a vegie stick or home-made cracker. This is also a really simple recipe to prepare and enjoy with kids.

1 large pomegranate

520 g (1 lb 2½ oz/2 cups) full-fat plain sheep's milk yoghurt, chilled

2 spring onions (scallions), finely chopped

small handful coriander (cilantro) leaves, finely chopped, plus extra sprigs to garnish

pinch of sea salt

¼ teaspoon ground cumin

1 tablespoon lemon juice

mint sprigs, to serve

Sesame Flat Bread (page 254), to serve

Cut the pomegranate in half and gently scoop out the seeds in segments, being careful not to break them. Pull the seeds off the yellow pithy membrane.

In a medium bowl, combine the yoghurt, spring onion, coriander, salt and cumin, and mix well to combine. Add the lemon juice and check the seasoning. Gently fold in the pomegranate seeds, reserving some for a garnish.

Transfer to a serving bowl, then garnish with the reserved pomegranate seeds and mint and coriander sprigs. Serve with the sesame flat bread.

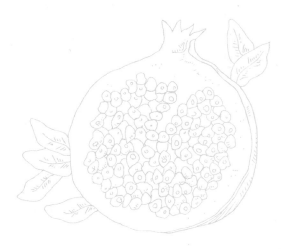

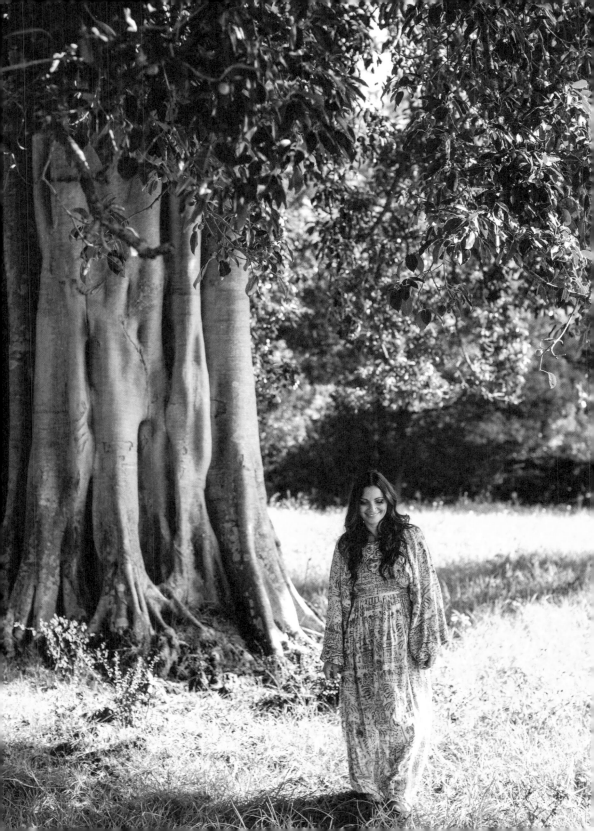

Quinoa tabouleh

{ *SERVES* 4 }

This wheat-free version of the healthy Middle Eastern dish is ready in minutes, and will bring superb freshness and nutrients. I love it as a super-easy fresh vegetarian side dish or light lunch. This version replaces the traditional burghul (bulgur) with gluten-free quinoa, which transforms it into a more filling and wholesome dish.

440 g (15½ oz/2 cups) cooked quinoa, cooled

¼ red onion, finely chopped

2 tomatoes, chopped

large handful flat-leaf (Italian) parsley, finely chopped

1 garlic clove, finely chopped

1½ tablespoons extra virgin olive oil

1 tablespoon lemon juice

pinch of sea salt

Mix together the quinoa, onion, tomato, parsley and garlic.

Whisk together the olive oil, lemon juice and salt in a small bowl. Pour over the salad and stir to combine.

Chicken pot pies

{ *SERVES* 4 }

Pies are one of my favourite ways to add comfort during the autumn and winter months. I feel a little leap of joy when I crack through the golden roof of flaky pastry and inhale the fragrant steam that emerges. Pies are also a handy way to use up extra vegies or herbs you have on hand and reduce food waste.

1 tablespoon extra virgin olive oil

1 garlic clove, crushed

1 brown onion, diced

2 boneless, skinless chicken breasts, diced

1 small sweet potato, peeled and diced

140 g (5 oz/1 cup) frozen peas, thawed

1 teaspoon dried parsley

1 teaspoon dried thyme

2 tablespoons gluten-free rice flour

500 ml (17 fl oz/2 cups) home-made chicken stock

sea salt and freshly ground black pepper, to taste

2 sheets gluten-free filo pastry

Preheat the oven to 180°C (350°F) and grease four individual pie dishes.

Heat the olive oil in a large frying pan over medium heat. Fry the garlic and onion for 2–3 minutes, until slightly coloured. Add the chicken and cook to seal on all sides, then add the sweet potato and cook for 10 minutes, stirring frequently. Add the peas and herbs, and cook for 3–4 minutes, stirring occasionally.

Mix the rice flour with a little of the stock in a small bowl, then pour into the pan with the remaining stock and stir through. Bring to the boil, then reduce the heat to low and simmer, stirring, for 10 minutes, or until the liquid thickens. Season with salt and pepper.

Divide the mixture between the prepared pie dishes. Stack the filo sheets and cut into quarters. Cover each pie dish with the pastry, trimming as necessary and tucking the edges inside the dish. Bake on the middle shelf of the oven for 40 minutes, or until the pastry is golden.

Gooey baklava

{ *MAKES ABOUT 12* }

I think baklava has to be one of the most insanely addictive sweet treats going around. There's something about the combo of dense nuts, light crunchy filo pastry and the blissful sweetness of fragrant syrup that sends me into a frenzy. This wholefood version is honestly one of the most delicious recipes in my repertoire, and nearly always causes an awkward pause as two people negotiate who will take the last piece.

360 g (12¾ oz/3 cups) finely chopped walnuts

1 teaspoon ground cinnamon

grated zest of 1 orange

250 g (9 oz) butter, melted

20 sheets gluten-free filo pastry

1 teaspoon sesame seeds

Honey syrup

250 ml (9 fl oz/1 cup) filtered water

150 g (5½ oz/1 cup) coconut sugar

180 g (6¼ oz/½ cup) rice malt syrup

1 cinnamon stick

½ teaspoon cloves

½ teaspoon grated orange zest

Preheat the oven to 175°C (345°F) and grease a shallow 20 cm (8 inch) square baking tin.

In a medium bowl, mix the nuts, cinnamon and orange zest. Lay three sheets of filo in the prepared tin, then brush with melted butter. Scatter over 2–3 tablespoons of the nut mixture, then top with a sheet of filo. Continue with melted butter, nuts and single filo sheets until all the pastry has been used, ending with filo. Score the final layer in a diamond pattern, brush with melted butter, top with sesame seeds and tuck in the edges.

Bake for 20–25 minutes, until golden brown.

Meanwhile, prepare the honey syrup. Combine all the ingredients in a medium saucepan and bring to the boil over medium heat. Reduce the heat to low and simmer for 20 minutes. Strain, discarding the spices, pour over the baklava and leave for at least 10 minutes for the syrup to soak in. Cut along the score lines and serve.

Fig, hazelnut and goat's cheese tart

{ *SERVES 6* }

This tart is the perfect bring-along if you're invited to dinner and want to contribute a dessert with some wow factor. The roasted crunchy hazelnuts intermingle beautifully with the soft sweetness of roasted figs and a tangy edge of creamy goat's cheese. Yum! Figs are also considered an aphrodisiac.

55 g (2 oz) hazelnuts, roasted and chopped, plus extra to serve

2 sheets gluten-free shortcrust pastry

55 g (2 oz) unsalted butter

50 g (1¾ oz/⅓ cup) coconut sugar

½ teaspoon ground cinnamon

1 egg

150 g (5½ oz) goat's cheese

10 figs, halved

rice malt syrup, for drizzling (optional)

rosemary sprigs, to serve (optional)

Preheat the oven to 220°C (425°F) and line a baking tray with baking paper.

Grind the hazelnuts in a food processor. Carefully lay the pastry sheets side by side on the prepared tray overlapping them slightly and pressing down on the join. Press around gently with a knife to mark a 2 cm (¾ inch) border without going all the way through. Fold the edges over along the score mark.

In a medium bowl, mix the butter, ground hazelnuts, 2 tablespoons of the coconut sugar, and the cinnamon and egg, working it into a paste using a fork. Spread over the pastry, keeping the border clear. Crumble half the goat's cheese over the tart. Arrange the figs on top, then crumble over the remaining goat's cheese and scatter over the extra hazelnuts. Sprinkle the remaining coconut sugar over the top.

Bake for 12–15 minutes, until the pastry is puffy and golden. Serve topped with a drizzle of rice malt syrup and garnished with rosemary, if using.

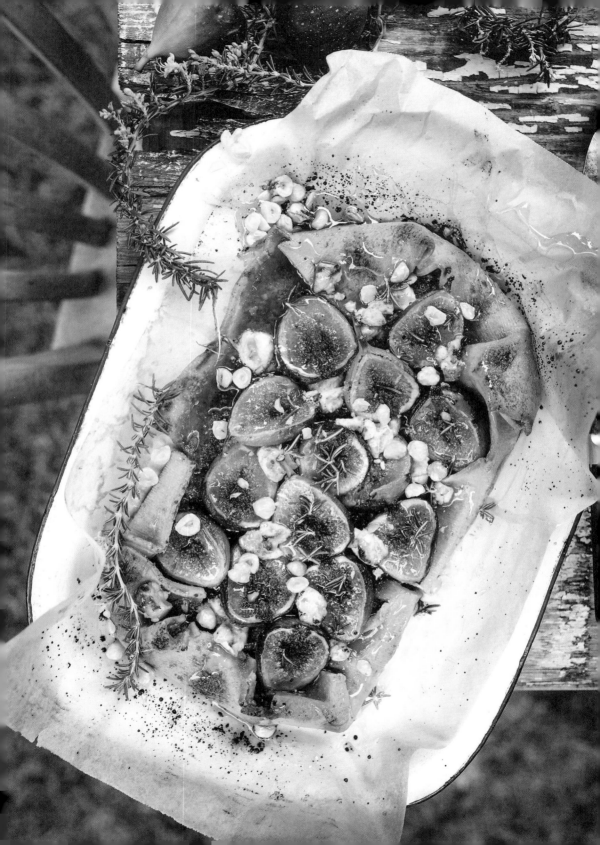

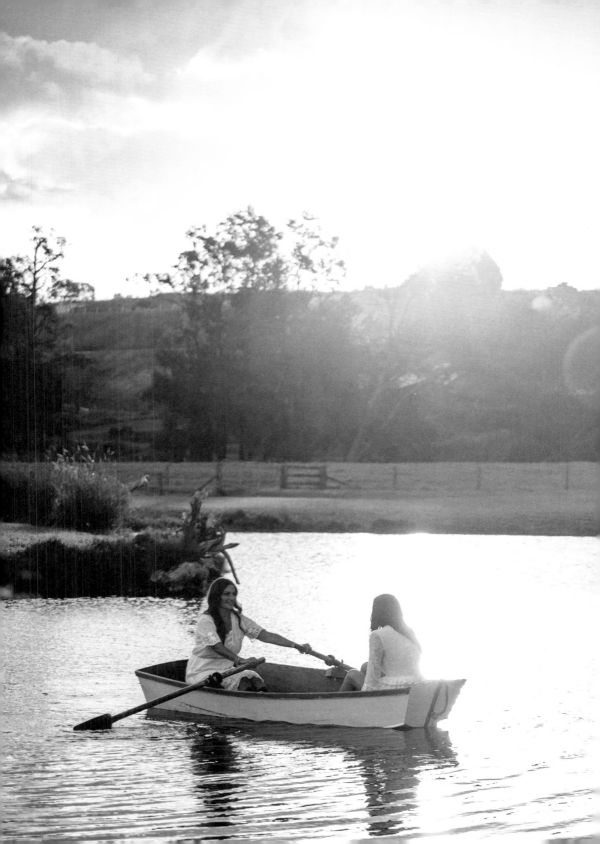

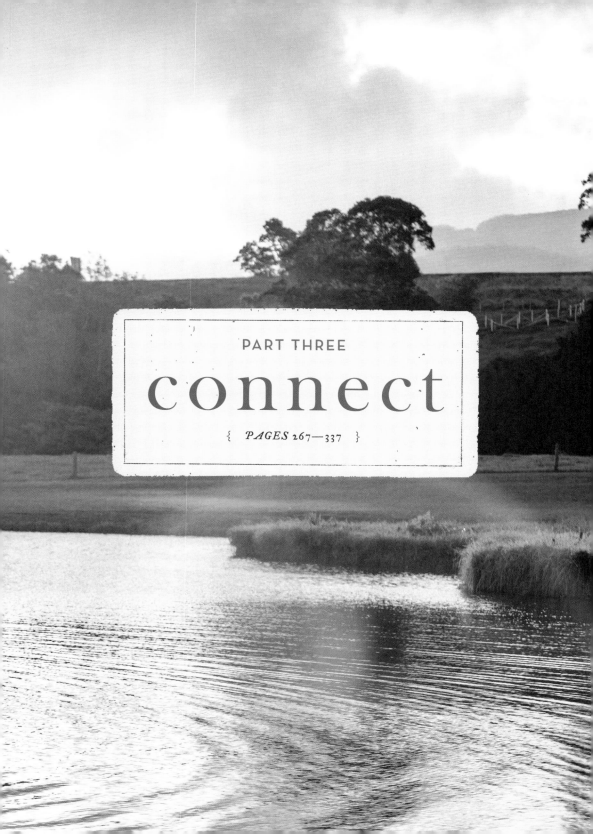

PART THREE

connect

{ *PAGES* 267—337 }

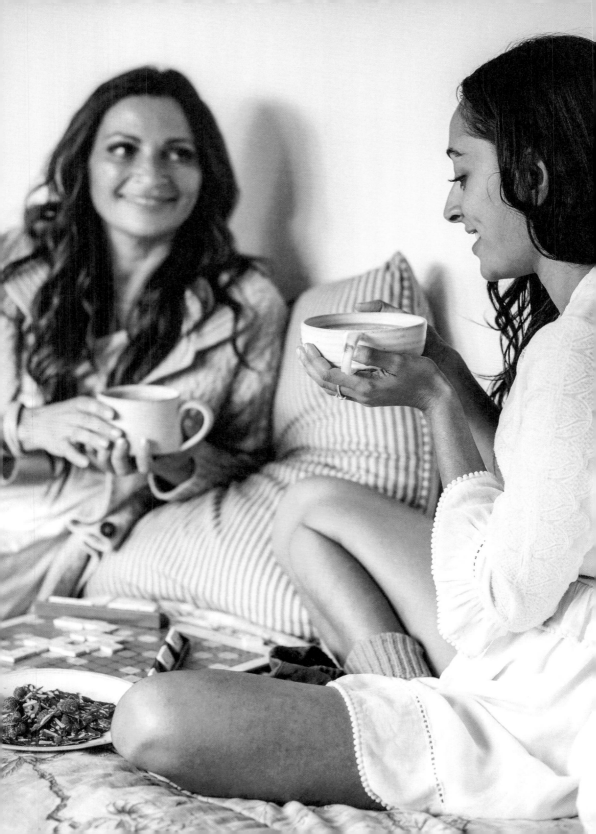

Joining the dots

In the last decade, science has been unveiling the fascinating connection between our mind and our body. Previously, we thought there were narrow cause-and-effect links between the food we ate and health outcomes, but we're now learning that our minds and thinking play an immensely important role in the way our physical body functions. These breakthroughs have come via the study of epigenetics (how genes are expressed), neuroplasticity, the vagus nerve, the microbiome and the brain.

Now let's go back to the concept of pleasure I introduced at the beginning of this book. We humans are programmed to seek pleasure and avoid pain. When we eat, we seek the pleasure of food and we avoid the pain of hunger. As the Institute for the Psychology of Eating in Boulder, Colorado, says, vitamin P (pleasure) is a vital factor in making our meals nutritionally complete and also plays a role in our metabolism. When we're turned on by our food, we turn on our metabolism. Studies from the University of Texas, for example, have revealed a strange phenomenon. When people aiming to lower their cholesterol through diet restriction were allowed to 'splurge' on foods such as milkshakes and fast food, their cholesterol didn't rise as expected. Studies from Sweden and Thailand on the cultural appreciation of foods have shown fascinating indications that significantly more iron is absorbed by cultural groups eating meals they naturally enjoy. This indicates a complex link between our psychological appreciation of a food and our uptake of nutrients from it.

So what does that mean for you and how do you apply it to a supercharged life? If you're experiencing a limited sense of enjoyment and pleasure when eating food, you might not be receiving the nutritional benefits you really crave. But there is a solution. Eat foods for the sake of genuine enjoyment rather than for some other agenda, such as a diet or a particular health outcome. Now how liberating and supercharging is that?

Finding freedom

Take a moment to think about your personal attitude to food.

UNHEALTHY VS HEALTHY

I'd encourage you, in the name of pleasure and freedom, to begin to depollute some of the unhelpful thinking you may have accumulated when it comes to food. This example of a 'thought swap' could help you on your way. I've included specific questions you can ask yourself and respond to honestly, to explore and possibly heal the negative emotions at the base of your thinking about food. Exploring these thoughts and answering the questions in a journal is a great way to acknowledge and address any unhealthy attitudes that could be stealing your joy and happiness.

UNHEALTHY THOUGHT: 'I really want to eat that piece of chocolate cake/other food but I'll get fat/sick/[some other fear].'

QUESTIONS FOR REFLECTION: Ask yourself:

1   Is my choice coming from a place of fear or freedom?

2   Can I say yes to this food and be free from guilt? Why/why not?

3   Can I say no to this food and be free from feelings of victimisation and deprivation? Why/why not?

4   What is my body really asking for right now?

5   Will this food bring me pleasure and enrich my life?

HEALTHY THOUGHTS: 'I acknowledge I have a desire for this particular food. I'm aware of my body and its needs.'

'I won't be guided by the fear of becoming fat/sick/[your other fear].'

'Whatever I choose to eat, I do so with ease, enjoyment and freedom from guilt.'

FINDING FOOD FREEDOM

Finding freedom in eating is primarily about creating a mindset that encourages you to cook and eat out of love for yourself and for life. If you're struggling to find motivation, write out a few of your favourite liberating words (or those below) and stick them up on your fridge or another area of your house where you'll be reminded of them daily. This will help you to maintain a balanced approach to eating for wellness and pleasure. Remember that if you can change your mind, you can change your life!

'So many people are afraid of food, afraid of their own appetite, afraid of experiencing pleasure from food, afraid that if they start to eat something they'll never stop. Such fears around food and body point to a powerful life lesson: learning to trust. Trust in your body, trust your choices, and trust that even when you make a mistake, you can return to a place of self-compassion and begin again.' — *Emily Rosen*

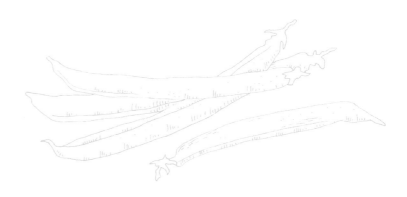

Moving away from fear

We live in a nutrition-obsessed world, particularly in the blogosphere and social media realms. Many bloggers and online wellbeing entrepreneurs, including me, have shared their stories of how good nutrition caused a positive transformation or healing experience in their lives. When we feel the benefits of eating healthy food, we want to shout it from the rooftops, and with good reason: our bodies will always welcome real, fresh nutrient-dense foods. Nutrition just works.

But there can be complications. We all have a unique and incredibly fascinating relationship with food. You may already be passionate about eating healthily, but perhaps your relationship with eating is somehow tainted by a body-image disorder, fear of gaining weight, emotional eating, chronic dieting, binge-eating, overeating, or some other challenge that makes the everyday, natural act of feeding yourself a battle.

Even if your plate is regularly full of organic, green, beautiful food, you can still have a niggling lack of peace within yourself. Perhaps underlying your love of filling your body with nutritious food is really a fear of dying, or a fear of losing control of your health, your beauty, your energy or your capacity to maintain your high-powered life, or maybe some other emotional issue is at work. Maybe healthy eating has become more of a burden than a blessing due to the underlying emotional motivations.

Another barrier to enjoying food is the constant avalanche of conflicting information from the internet and media regarding what's healthy and what's dangerous to eat. It seems we can't win. One day a particular superfood will be in the spotlight, and the next day it's slandered as dangerous. Even the 'experts' can't agree.

Nutrition is an incredibly complex topic, and it can be difficult to stay confident in our choices when there is a cascade of information from research laboratories. To remain truly peaceful in your relationship with food, and to live a supercharged life, your motivation must extend beyond what's printed in the media.

I believe that in this era of clean-eating, kale-smoothie obsession, we've lost our pure enjoyment of food. We've become so afraid of gluten, sugar, fructose, dairy, meat, unfiltered water and grains that many of us have eliminated them completely from our diet with no balance or moderation. Do any of these thoughts sound familiar?

- 'I'd love to try a bit of that spelt sourdough, but aren't grains supposed to kill my brain and cause Alzheimer's disease?'

- 'That yoghurt looks divine, but will dairy give me cellulite and an autoimmune condition?'

- 'I'd love to have some of that mango, but will that extra fructose have a negative effect on my body?'

If these types of thoughts dwell in your head constantly, the chances are your attitude to food has shifted from joy to rules and restrictions.

While some foods can be genuinely harmful for some people, the reality is that not everyone responds to food in the same way. I know people who have lived to 100 on a lifetime of bread, cream, meat and a good few decades of cigarettes, and they enjoyed greater health than people who obsess over their daily shot of spirulina. There has to be more to the picture, and there has to be balance.

I believe food is on this earth to be enjoyed and we think about it way too much. Fair enough, if you know you're not feeling your most vibrant self when you eat a certain way, seek out a professional to help you find a diet that works best for you. But don't throw the baby out with the bathwater. Avoiding a natural food out of fear, 'just in case' it might cause an autoimmunity issue, an imbalance of gut bacteria or cancer down the track is not living. It's crippling, and it's the opposite of a supercharged approach.

My greatest hope is that this book will help to reignite your love of commonsense eating and free you from the fear of food.

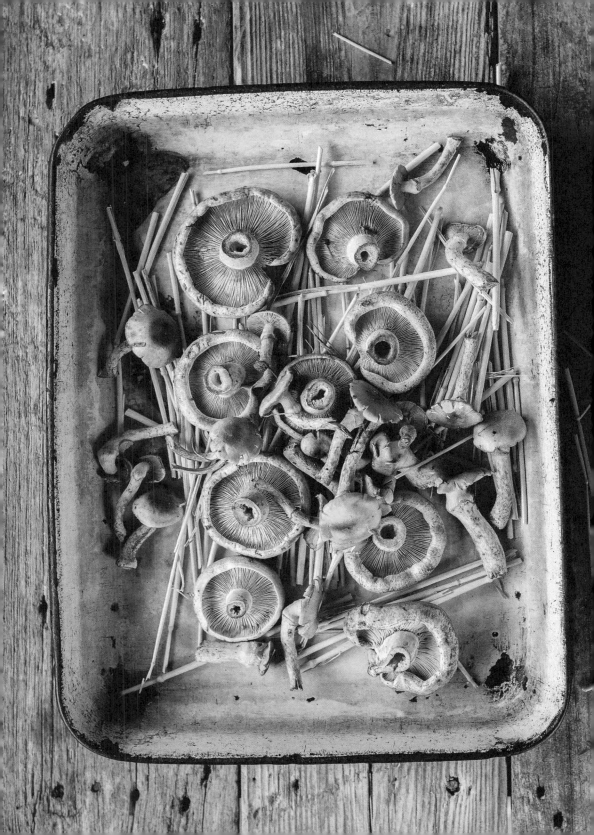

Commonsense eating

The everyday act of consuming food should never bring you a feeling of captivity or worry. In a supercharged life, food is to be enjoyed and savoured. Here, we walk to the unforced rhythms that come with a commonsense attitude towards food and a balanced approach to eating. Letting go of a rule-bound approach to eating will bring you a sense of freedom, but still allow you to commit to food choices that equate to vibrant health and longevity - and a life fully lived.

I've pulled together a list here of the basic commonsense eating guidelines I live by. Instead of being motivated by the fear of negative consequences, why not try to implement one or more of these in your life?

1 ## Eat mostly plants
Despite the vast differences in doctrine between the mainstream and alternative nutrition experts, the one thing we can all agree on is that eating plant foods is really good. I like to ensure that plant foods - such as nuts, seeds, fruits, grains (brown rice, oats, quinoa, buckwheat), fruits, sea vegetables, herbs and spices - make up the majority of my diet, with the greatest emphasis on seasonal vegetables and especially greens. I still enjoy animal products such as meat, eggs, fish, cheese, butter and ghee, but in smaller quantities.

2 ## Avoid processed foods where you can
Industrially produced foods that your ancestors wouldn't comprehend are best eaten in small amounts. Any ingredient with a number, or a name that doesn't register as 'food' when you read it, probably *isn't* food. Stick to things that are foods, in as natural a state as possible. If a laboratory or factory has done most of the preparation, it's probably better to leave it on the supermarket shelf.

3 ## Live by the 80:20 rule
Sticking to your nutritional values 80 per cent of the time will allow you a healthy margin where you can say yes to the chocolate cake at your friends' birthday parties, or enjoy a big slab of pizza as you travel through Naples. There are food opportunities in life that just can't be ignored or turned down.

Don't be that killjoy. Allowing yourself the space to stray from your regular nourishing eating habits will help you not to take yourself too seriously, and will bring freedom to your social food situations. Twenty per cent indulgence won't do you any harm if you're otherwise healthy.

4 **Balance out your eating**
Eating is all about balance. If you've been out of your normal routine while at work or on holidays and found you've overindulged in a specific food, spend the next few days nourishing yourself back to homoeostasis (metabolic balance) with the foods you've been missing. If you've spent a few days eating lots of starchy, cooked foods, for example, it might be a good idea to spend a couple of days eating some raw and lighter foods through vegie juices, salads and vegetable soups.

5 **Take an Ayurvedic approach**
Traditional Ayurvedic medicine teaches us that we attain health when we eat a practical balance of different types of foods from the taste categories of bitter, sweet, sour, salty, astringent and pungent. Having a varied diet of different tastes, eating seasonally, and ensuring the right balance of cooked and cold foods helps the nervous system recognise nourishment. You can work out your ideal Ayurvedic eating plan by determining your *dosha*, which will help you eat in a commonsense way for your unique body type.

6 **Choose quality over quantity**
This is especially true with animal products. Overall, try to invest in better-quality food that's chemical-free or organic. Shop at local farmers' markets rather than supermarkets if possible. With animal products, look for organic or 100 per cent grass-fed and grass-finished. It's better to enjoy smaller amounts of quality food than gorging on food that's cheap and of lower quality.

7 **Eat mindfully**
Do what the French do and make an occasion of your meal, even if it's just morning or afternoon tea. Unplug, turn off the TV, sit at the table, use proper dinnerware, eat with friends and family, and give thanks. Tune in to all your senses and pay attention to enjoying and savouring each glorious mouthful. Enjoy the following morning and afternoon tea delights.

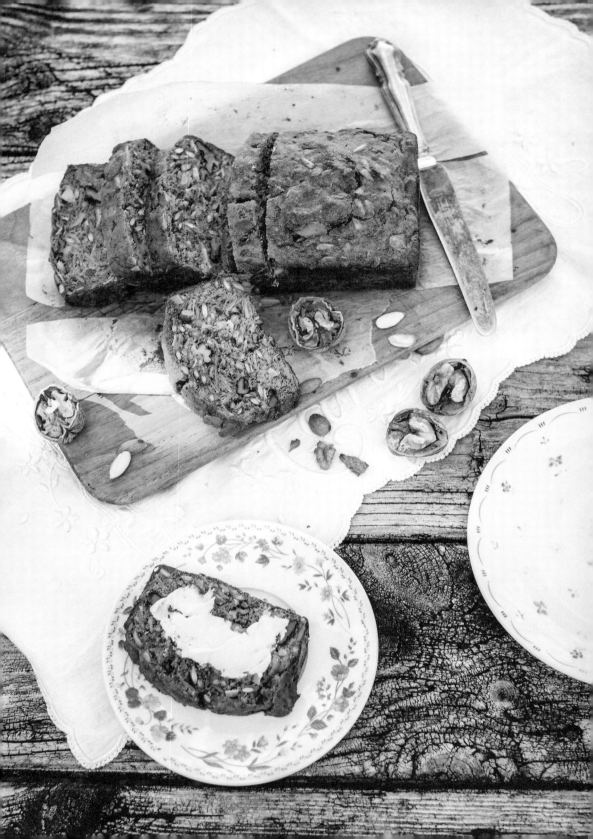

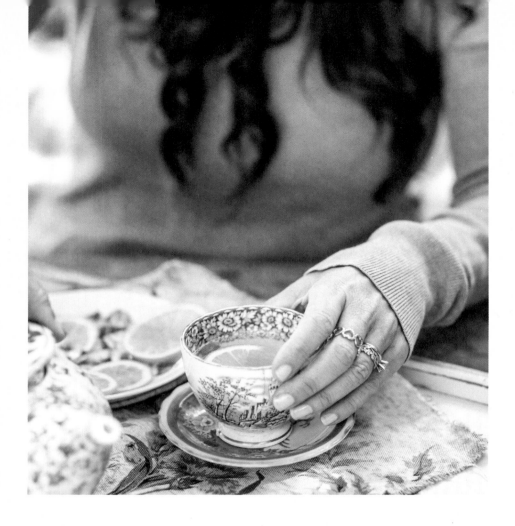

Warming ginger, cardamom and lime tea

{ *SERVES* 1 }

375 ml (13 fl oz/1½ cups)
  filtered water

1 teaspoon grated fresh ginger
  or ¼ teaspoon ground ginger

1 tablespoon lemon juice

1 teaspoon lime zest

1 tablespoon grated lime juice

2 cardamom pods, pounded,
  or ½ teaspoon ground
  cardamom

6 drops liquid stevia, or to taste

In a small saucepan over medium heat, combine the water, ginger, lemon juice, and lime zest and juice. Bring to the boil, stirring. Remove from the heat and add the cardamom, then cover and allow the tea to steep for 3–4 minutes. Add the stevia and enjoy.

'Cheesy' tomato and basil braids

{ *MAKES* 8 }

1 sheet gluten-free puff pastry

1 egg, lightly beaten

200 g (7 oz/1 cup) chopped
   tomatoes

20 g (³/₄ oz/¹/₄ cup) nutritional
   yeast flakes

small handful basil leaves,
   shredded

Preheat the oven to 210°C (410°F) and line
a baking tray with baking paper.

Lay the pastry on a clean work surface,
brush with the egg and cut into 1 cm (¹/₂ inch)
strips. Join three of the strips at one end,
then braid (plait) them together. Repeat with
the remaining strips. Lay the braids on the
prepared baking tray.

In a medium bowl, combine the tomatoes,
yeast flakes and basil. Place teaspoonfuls of
the mixture in each depression in the braids
and bake for 10–15 minutes, until puffy and
golden. They will keep in an airight container
for 3–4 days.

*Note: For a photo of these braids, see
pages 336–37.*

Spiced hazelnut and orange biscuits

{ *MAKES 6 LARGE OR 12 SMALL* }

75 g (2³/₄ oz) unsalted butter,
   softened

175 g (6 oz) coconut sugar

1 large egg

175 g (6 oz/1³/₄ cups) almond
   meal or ground cashews

¹/₂ teaspoon bicarbonate of
   soda (baking soda)

grated zest of 1 orange

¹/₂ teaspoon freshly grated
   nutmeg

¹/₂ teaspoon ground cinnamon

50 g (1³/₄ oz/¹/₃ cup) hazelnuts,
   roughly chopped

Preheat the oven to 180°C (350°F). Line
a baking tray with baking paper.

Beat the butter and coconut sugar in a medium
bowl until creamy, then beat in the egg. Fold in
the remaining ingredients with a spoon. Drop
spoonfuls of the mixture on the prepared
baking tray, leaving a 2.5 cm (1 inch) gap
between them.

Bake for 12–15 minutes, until just golden but
still soft in the middle. Cool completely on
a wire rack then store in an airtight container
for 3–4 days.

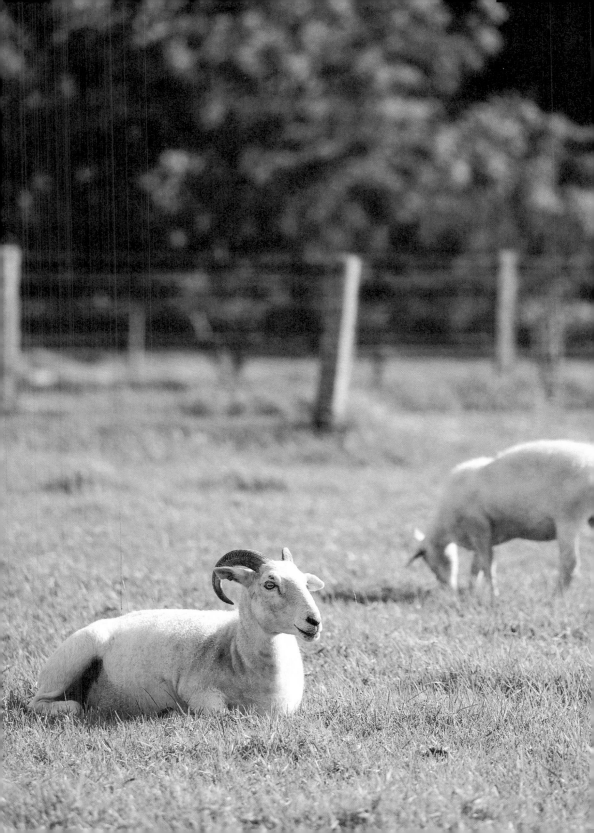

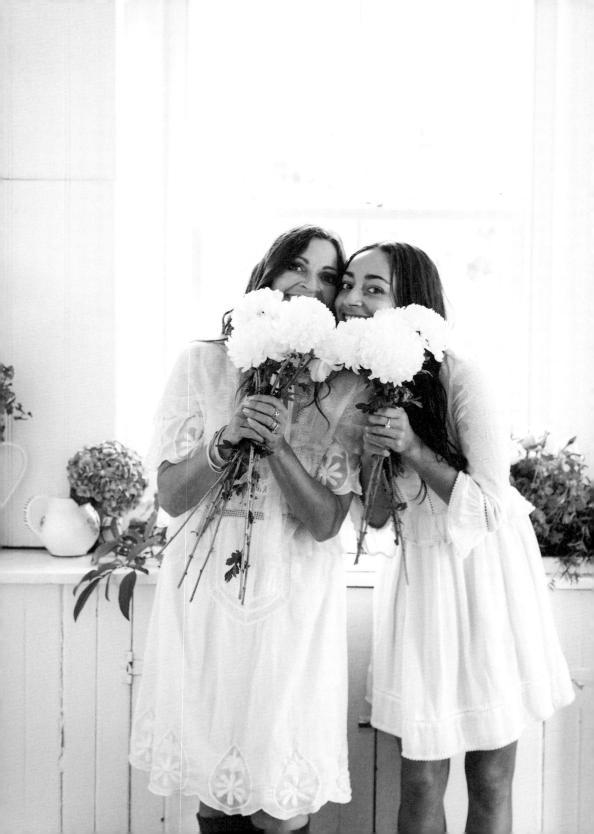

Chocolate cravings

{ *SERVES 6* }

The world would be a sad place without chocolate, and I have no concern about indulging regularly if it's made with love from real ingredients. The two ways of using this chocolate sauce are real winners: Chocolate-coated Strawberries are perfect for a light post-dinner sweet craving, and Chocolate Mint Discs are a beautiful reinvention of the after-dinner mint.

Chocolate sauce

125 ml (4 fl oz/^{1}/$_2$ cup) coconut oil

90 g (3^1/$_4$ oz) coconut butter

180 g (6^1/$_4$ oz/^{1}/$_2$ cup) rice malt syrup

2 tablespoons raw cacao powder

1 teaspoon alcohol-free vanilla extract

For Chocolate-coated strawberries

6 strawberries, hulled and chilled in the fridge

For Chocolate mint discs

20 g (^{3}/$_4$ oz/^{1}/$_3$ cup) coconut flakes

50 g (1^3/$_4$ oz/^{1}/$_3$ cup) raw cashews

2 tablespoons melted coconut butter

2–3 tablespoons rice malt syrup

1 teaspoon peppermint essence

pinch of sea salt

To make the chocolate sauce, melt the coconut oil and coconut butter in a bowl sitting over – but not touching – a bowl of boiling water. Whisk together until they are mostly melted and warmed through to room temperature (see tip).

Place the remaining sauce ingredients in a food processor. Add the coconut oil and coconut butter mixture and blend until combined. Chill until ready to use for a more solid consistency.

For the chocolate strawberries option, sit the strawberries in an ice-cube tray. Pour chilled chocolate sauce over the strawberries and refrigerate until set.

For the chocolate mint discs option, line a baking tray with baking paper. Blend all the ingredients in a food processor until smooth. Spread the mint layer out on the prepared baking tray and press flat using your hands. Cut out discs with a cookie cutter and freeze for about 30 minutes, until set. Dip each disc in the chocolate sauce and refrigerate until the chocolate is set.

SUPERCHARGED TIP

Please don't microwave your oil and butter or heat them on the stovetop. You'll destroy the good antimicrobial properties in the oil and it won't blend in well with the cacao powder. If you end up with a watery mess, you overheated the coconut oil and butter.

Banana, raspberry and chia seed muffins

{ *MAKES* 12 }

300 g (10½ oz/3 cups) almond meal

35 g (1¼ oz/½ cup) shredded coconut

1 tablespoon ground cinnamon

1 teaspoon vanilla powder

1 teaspoon gluten-free baking powder

35 g (1¼ oz/¼ cup) chia seeds

3 eggs

40 g (1½ oz) butter or 2 tablespoons coconut oil, melted

2 tablespoons coconut milk

360 g (12¾ oz/1½ cups/about 3½) mashed overripe bananas

125 g (4½ oz/1 cup) raspberries

pinch of sea salt

Preheat the oven to 180°C (350°F) and line a 12 × 80 ml (2½ fl oz/⅓ cup) hole muffin tray with paper cases.

In a large bowl, mix together the almond meal, coconut, cinnamon, vanilla powder, baking powder and chia seeds.

In a separate bowl, whisk the eggs with the butter and coconut milk until combined. Fold in the mixed dry ingredients. Fold in the banana, then gently fold in the raspberries, reserving 12 to decorate.

Fill the muffin cases to three-quarters, then halve the reserved raspberries and place one on each muffin.

Bake for 15–20 minutes, until golden brown on top. Cool in the tin for 5 minutes, then transfer to a wire rack to cool completely.

Royal sandwich biscuits

{ *MAKES 8-10* }

The humble bickie (cookie) is a salve to the emotions as much as to the tastebuds, and these royal sandwich biscuits are the cream of the crop. Biscuits are the ultimate sweet comfort food when dunked in a steaming cup of tea, and this simple invitation to a friend is part of the fabric of our society - it's one of the easiest forms of hospitality! In an age of fleeting fads and virtual reality, deep down we value things that are real and enduring. Coconut biscuits sandwiched around a chocolate filling is a combo Aussies have enjoyed for years.

Coconut biscuits

100 g (3½ oz/1 cup) almond meal

30 g (1 oz/¼ cup) coconut flour

1 teaspoon bicarbonate of soda (baking soda)

¼ teaspoon salt

110 g (3¾ oz) coconut oil or unsalted butter, melted

110 g (3¾ oz/¾ cup) coconut sugar

100 g (3½ oz/⅓ cup) almond butter

1½ teaspoons vanilla powder

1 large egg, lightly beaten

Chocolate filling

80 g (2¾ oz) good-quality chocolate, broken into pieces

80 ml (2½ fl oz/⅓ cup) coconut cream

1 teaspoon vanilla powder

pinch of sea salt

To make the chocolate filling, melt the chocolate in a small saucepan over low heat then stir in the remaining ingredients. Let it stand for a minute or two, then stir and set aside to cool until it thickens.

Preheat the oven to 175°C (345°F) and line a baking tray with baking paper.

In a medium bowl, mix the almond meal, coconut flour, bicarbonate of soda and salt.

In a large bowl, beat the coconut oil and coconut sugar for about 1 minute. Stir in the almond butter, vanilla powder and egg until well mixed.

Fold the almond meal mixture into the egg mixture, then refrigerate for 30 minutes. Roll the dough into 16-20 balls, place on the prepared baking tray with at least 2.5 cm (1 inch) between them, and press each one down with a spatula.

Bake for 12-15 minutes, until golden, then cool completely on the baking tray. They'll be soft in the middle, but will harden as they cool.

Once cool, spread 1 tablespoon of filling on half the biscuits. Place a second biscuit on top, then leave for a minute or two for the chocolate to set. Store in an airtight container in the fridge for 4-5 days.

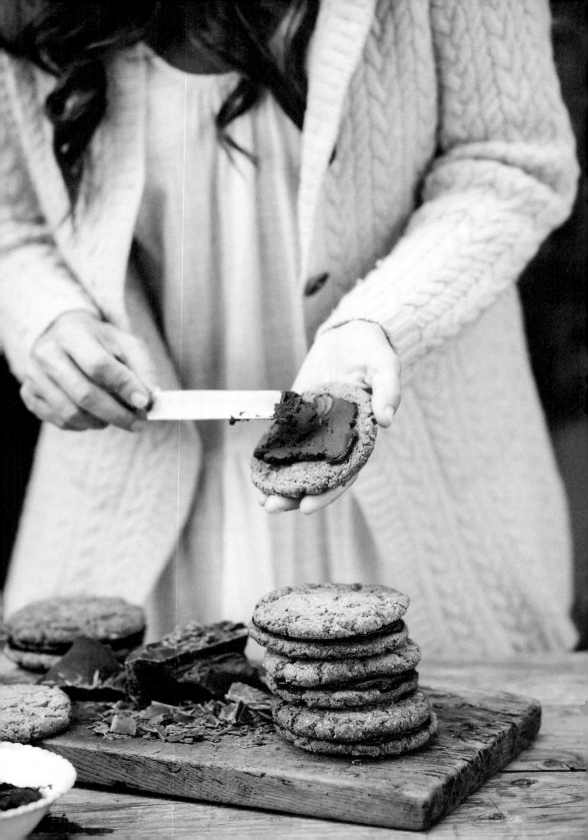

Raw chocolate tart with berry sauce

{ *SERVES 6* }

A trusty blender makes this showstopper cake so easy you could almost make it blindfolded. You can whiz together this magnificent dessert in about 15 minutes – the rest of the magic is done in the fridge. This cake just screams romance, and is a gorgeous act of love at the end of a Valentine's Day feast, or to light up a girlfriend's birthday or baby shower celebration.

edible flowers and fresh berries, and mint leaves (optional), to serve

Base

155 g (5½ oz/1 cup) raw cashews

65 g (2¼ oz/1 cup) shredded coconut

¼ teaspoon stevia powder

60 ml (2 fl oz/¼ cup) lemon juice

25 g (1 oz) coconut butter, melted

Filling

6 very ripe avocados, peeled

250 ml (9 fl oz/1 cup) almond or coconut milk

180 g (6¼ oz/½ cup) rice malt syrup or your sweetener of choice

80 g (2¾ oz/¾ cup) raw cacao powder

70 g (2½ oz/½ cup) chia seeds

3 teaspoons alcohol-free vanilla extract

Berry sauce

325 g (11½ oz/2½ cups) mixed fresh or frozen berries

2 tablespoons coconut nectar or rice malt syrup

1 teaspoon alcohol-free vanilla extract

Grease an 18 cm (7 inch) loose-based flan (tart) tin.

To make the base, process the cashews and coconut in a blender until finely chopped. Transfer to a medium bowl and stir in the remaining ingredients, adding a little filtered water if necessary – the mixture should be stiff and hold together while not being too crumbly. Using your hands, mould into a dough and press into the prepared tin. Freeze for 20 minutes to set.

Blend all the filling ingredients in a high-speed blender or food processor for 30 seconds or until smooth and creamy. Pour over the base and smooth the top using a spatula. Refrigerate for 1–2 hours, until set.

To make the berry sauce, whiz all the ingredients in a blender or food processor.

Top the cake with the berry sauce, and serve decorated with edible flowers, fresh berries and mint leaves, if using.

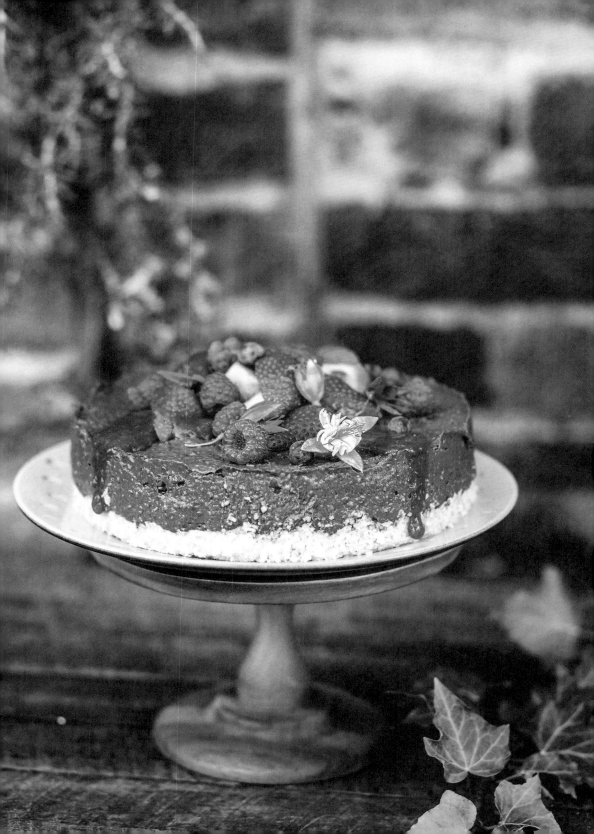

Vegan cheese platter

I often crave a creamy cheese platter rather than a sweet dessert after dinner. But dairy can leave some people feeling weighed down and bloated rather than satisfied. I love this vegan cheese platter served with some organic grapes, sundried tomatoes, home-made crackers and a glass of your favourite tipple. Why not try my Fennel and Poppy Seed Crackers (page 250), Sesame Flat Bread (page 254) or Turmeric Sesame Crackers (page 255)?

Cashew cheese

{ *MAKES ABOUT* 250 G [9 OZ] }

If you are a vegan, you will of course make this with agar-agar rather than gelatine.

250 ml (9 fl oz/1 cup) filtered water

1½ teaspoons powdered gelatine or agar-agar

50 g (1¾ oz/⅓ cup) raw cashews, soaked in filtered water for 2 hours

1½ tablespoons nutritional yeast flakes

1½ teaspoons tapioca flour

1½ tablespoons lemon juice

small pinch of ground turmeric

sea salt, to taste

Grease a medium (about 400 ml/14 fl oz capacity) ramekin.

Pour half of the water into a small saucepan, sprinkle the gelatine over and set aside.

Drain the cashews and dry them with paper towel. In a food processor, blend the cashews with the nutritional yeast flakes, tapioca flour, lemon juice and turmeric. Add salt to taste and the remaining water to make a smooth paste.

Add the cashew mixture to the gelatine and water in the saucepan and bring to the boil over medium–low heat, stirring often, until the mixture has a thick pancake-batter-like consistency.

Pour into the prepared ramekin and refrigerate for about 1 hour, until set. Carefully remove the round from the ramekin. The cheese will have a softer consistency than hard cheese, but can be crumbled.

It will keep in the fridge for up to 3 days.

Baked almond feta

{ *MAKES ABOUT* 200 G [7 OZ] }

150 g (5½ oz/1½ cups) almond meal, or blanched almonds soaked for 2 hours in filtered water

375 ml (13 fl oz/1½ cups) filtered water

60 ml (2 fl oz/¼ cup) lemon juice

2 garlic cloves, peeled

25 g (1 oz/⅓ cup) nutritional yeast flakes

pinch of ground turmeric

1 teaspoon sea salt, or to taste

Line a colander with muslin (cheesecloth).

Whiz all the ingredients in a blender until creamy and very smooth, stopping to scrape down the side if necessary.

Spoon the mixture into the prepared colander, pressing it down, then take the muslin edges, pull them together and secure the top with an elastic band. Sit the colander over a bowl and refrigerate for 12 hours or overnight.

Preheat the oven to 160°C (315°F) and line a baking tray with baking paper

Undo the muslin and turn the round of almond feta out onto the prepared baking tray, smooth rounded side up. Bake for 40-50 minutes, until slightly golden and cracked. It should be firm to the touch.

Cool, then store in an airtight container in the fridge for up to 2 weeks. The flavour improves with age!

Probiotic cheese

{ *MAKES ABOUT* 300 G [10½ OZ] }

This cheesy recipe was created by Marc from Back 2 Earth, a raw vegan health retreat and farm stay in Berry, New South Wales, where I had a wonderful visit. He's a whiz when it comes to vegan cheeses.

310 g (11 oz/2 cups) raw cashews, soaked in filtered water for 2 hours

½ garlic clove, peeled

contents of 4 probiotic capsules

pinch of sea salt

Blend all the ingredients in a high-speed blender. Scoop into a bowl or mould lined with plastic wrap, cover with the overhanging plastic, leave in a warm place for 2 days, then refrigerate for 48 hours.

VARIATION

For blue cheese, mix ½ cup of the probiotic cheese mixture with 2 tablespoons spirulina powder or a crushed spirulina tablet before setting in the mould.

Almond parmesan

{ *MAKES ABOUT* 150 G [5½ OZ] }

Sprinkle on pizzas, soups, salads or spiralised noodles.

155 g (5½ oz/1 cup) blanched almonds

2 tablespoons nutritional yeast flakes

1 teaspoon garlic powder

½ teaspoon sea salt

Pulse all the ingredients in a food processor until crumbly.

Thyme and cranberry cheese log

{ *MAKES ABOUT* 450 G [1 LB] }

310 g (11 oz/2 cups) raw cashews, soaked in filtered water for 2 hours

60 ml (2 fl oz/¼ cup) lemon juice

2 tablespoons nutritional yeast flakes

1 tablespoon coconut oil

2 teaspoons apple cider vinegar

1 teaspoon dried thyme

¾ teaspoon sea salt

¼ teaspoon freshly ground black pepper

65 g (2¼ oz/½ cup) slivered almonds

75 g (2¾ oz/½ cup) dried cranberries, roughly chopped

1 teaspoon dried herbs (e.g. thyme, oregano and basil) (optional)

Drain and rinse the cashews then blend all the ingredients except the slivered almonds, dried cranberries and herbs in a food processor until very smooth. Be patient and scrape down the sides as necessary.

Spoon the mixture onto a sheet of plastic wrap and wrap the cheese, twisting the ends and using your hands to make a log shape before squaring off the ends. Refrigerate for 6 hours or overnight.

When ready to serve, remove the cheese from the wrap. Scatter the almonds and cranberries over the wrap, then carefully roll the log over it, pressing the fruit and nuts into the log. Sprinkle over the dried herbs, if using.

Coconut scones with strawberry jam

{ *MAKES* 8–10 }

Coconut scones

150 g (5½ oz/1 cup) gluten-free plain (all-purpose) flour, plus extra for dusting

80 g (2¾ oz/½ cup) white rice flour

2 teaspoons gluten-free baking powder

25 g (1 oz/¼ cup) almond meal, plus 1 tablespoon extra

pinch of sea salt

185 ml (6 fl oz/¾ cup) coconut milk

Coconut 'Yoghurt' (page 195) or whipped coconut cream, to serve

Strawberry jam

500 g (1 lb 2 oz/3⅓ cups) strawberries, hulled and halved

90 g (3¼ oz/¼ cup) rice malt syrup

1 teaspoon alcohol-free vanilla extract

2 tablespoons white chia seeds

To make the strawberry jam, combine the strawberries, rice malt syrup and vanilla in a medium heavy-based saucepan over medium heat and bring to the boil. Stir for 20 minutes, until the consistency is thick and the berries have broken down. While still hot, pour into a 500 ml (17 fl oz/2 cup) sterilised screw-top jar. Stir in the chia seeds, seal the jar tightly, cool, then store in the fridge. It will keep for 2 weeks.

Preheat the oven to 220°C (425°F) and line a baking tray with baking paper.

Mix the flours, baking powder, almond meal and salt in a large bowl and make a well in the middle. Pour the coconut milk into the well and mix to form a dough.

Turn the dough onto a floured work surface, press into a sausage shape and cut into rounds. Place these on the prepared baking tray and bake for 10 minutes, or until they are cooked through.

Serve on the day of making, with the strawberry jam and coconut 'yoghurt' or whipped coconut cream.

Zesty coconut slice

{ *SERVES 6* }

Base

100 g (3½ oz) unsalted butter, softened

75 g (2¾ oz/½ cup) coconut sugar

1 egg, lightly beaten

60 g (2¼ oz/¾ cup) teff flour

25 g (1 oz/¼ cup) desiccated coconut

Lemon curd

50 g (1¾ oz) unsalted butter, diced

75 g (2¾ oz/½ cup) coconut sugar

1 egg, whisked

2 teaspoons grated lemon zest

60 ml (2 fl oz/¼ cup) lemon juice

Coconut topping

2 eggs, lightly beaten

75 g (2¾ oz/½ cup) coconut sugar

195 g (6¾ oz/3 cups) shredded coconut

Preheat the oven to 180°C (350°F). Grease a 15 × 30 cm (6 × 12 inch) baking tin with a lip and line it with baking paper.

To make the base, beat the butter and coconut sugar until creamy. Add the egg and beat until just combined. Fold in the teff flour and desiccated coconut. Spoon the mixture into the prepared tin and smooth the surface. Bake for 15 minutes, or until golden. Set aside to cool.

To make the lemon curd, melt the butter in a small saucepan over low heat with the coconut sugar, egg, lemon zest and juice, and whisk to combine. Cook for 5 minutes, whisking constantly, until the mixture starts to thicken. Remove from the heat and set aside to cool. It will thicken even more as it cools.

Remove the base from the oven and spread the curd over the top.

For the coconut topping, whisk the eggs and coconut sugar in a bowl, then fold in the shredded coconut. Press the topping onto the curd then bake for 15–20 minutes, until the coconut is lightly golden.

Allow to cool before cutting into pieces.

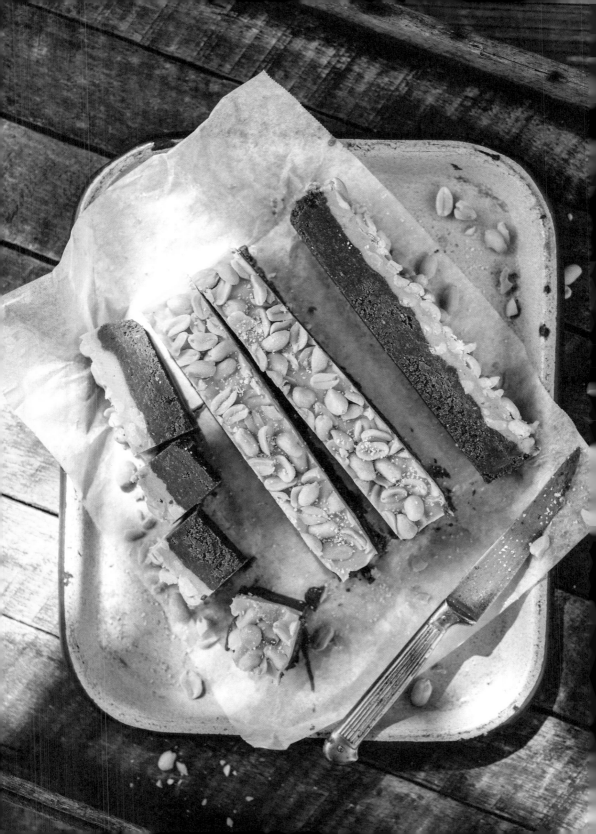

Layered salted caramel peanut fudge

{ *SERVES* 4–6 }

This is one of my favourite freezer desserts, and I like to keep it ready to grab at a moment's notice. A decadent delight, it homes in on the irresistible flavour combo of caramel and sea salt. The unique peanutty edge makes it fulfilling for adults with a cuppa, but also brings plenty of happiness to little kids.

Fudge

270 g (9½ oz/1 cup) almond butter

80 ml (2½ fl oz/⅓ cup) extra virgin coconut oil, melted

90 g (3¼ oz/¼ cup) rice malt syrup

30 g (1 oz/¼ cup) raw cacao powder

1 teaspoon alcohol-free vanilla extract

½ teaspoon Celtic sea salt

Salted caramel and peanut

90 g (3¼ oz/¼ cup) rice malt syrup

2 tablespoons cashew butter or other nut butter

2 tablespoons coconut oil

sea salt, to taste

35 g (1¼ oz/⅓ cup) roasted salted peanuts

Line a 12 × 18 cm (4½ × 7 inch) baking tin with baking paper.

To make the fudge layer, whiz the almond butter and coconut oil in a food processor until smooth. Add the remaining ingredients and process until smooth and creamy. Spoon the mixture into the prepared tin to 3 cm (1¼ inches) deep and smooth the top with the back of a spoon or a spatula.

For the salted caramel and peanut layer, clean the food processor then process all the ingredients except the peanuts until the mixture has a caramel-like consistency.

Spoon the salted caramel over the fudge, smooth with the back of a spoon or a spatula, then scatter the peanuts over and press them in gently. Freeze for at least 1 hour before slicing and serving. If stored frozen for longer, it may need some time in the fridge to soften a little before serving.

Sprinkle with extra salt before serving, if you like.

Hummingbird cake

{ *MAKES ONE LOAF* }

Loaf

3 ripe bananas, mashed

4 eggs

480 g (1 lb 1 oz) fresh pineapple flesh, cut into chunks, or 480 g (1 lb 1 oz) tinned pineapple chunks

300 g (10½ oz/3 cups) almond meal

60 g (2¼ oz/⅔ cup) desiccated coconut

55 g (2 oz/¼ cup) coconut oil, melted

2 teaspoons gluten-free baking powder

1 teaspoon sea salt

1 teaspoon ground cinnamon

¼ teaspoon bicarbonate of soda (baking soda)

115 g (4 oz/1 cup) chopped raw pecans, plus extra to decorate

Icing

150 g (5½ oz) cream cheese or whipped coconut cream

grated zest and juice of 1 lemon

2 teaspoons rice malt syrup

Preheat the oven to 160°C (315°F) and line a 12 × 12 cm (4½ × 8½ inch) loaf (bar) tin with baking paper.

Mix the bananas and eggs in a food processor until well combined. Add the remaining ingredients except the pecans and process until thoroughly mixed. Fold in the pecans until evenly distributed.

Pour the mixture into the prepared tin and bake for 50–60 minutes, until a skewer inserted in the centre comes out clean. Cool in the tin for 15 minutes then cool completely on a wire rack.

When the cake is cooled, make the icing. Beat all the ingredients with an electric mixer until combined. Spread the icing on the cake and decorate with the extra pecans.

Store in an airtight container in the fridge for up to 6 days.

Blueberry upside-down cake

{ *MAKES ONE 22 CM [8½ INCH] CAKE* }

390 g (13¾ oz/2½ cups) blueberries

180 g (6¼ oz/½ cup) rice malt syrup

240 g (8½ oz/1½ cups) white rice flour

130 g (4½ oz/1 cup) tapioca flour

½ teaspoon bicarbonate of soda (baking soda)

1½ teaspoons gluten-free baking powder

½ teaspoon fine sea salt

3 eggs, separated

90 g (3¼ oz) butter or coconut oil, melted

1½ teaspoons alcohol-free vanilla extract

250 ml (9 fl oz/1 cup) almond milk

Preheat the oven to 180°C (350°F) and line a 22 cm (8½ inch) round cake tin with baking paper.

Lay the blueberries in a single layer in the tin, drizzle over half the rice malt syrup and then set aside.

Sift the flours, bicarbonate of soda, baking powder and salt into a large bowl. Set aside.

Beat two of the egg yolks in a bowl with an electric mixer until pale (save the remaining yolk for another recipe). Add the butter, remaining rice malt syrup, vanilla and almond milk, and beat to combine. Fold in the flour mixture.

In a separate large bowl, beat the three egg whites with an electric mixer until stiff peaks form. Using a large spoon, gently fold the whites into the cake mixture. Spoon the mixture over the blueberries and smooth the top with the back of a spoon.

Bake for 40–45 minutes, until the top is golden and a skewer inserted in the centre comes out clean. Remove from the oven and cool in the tin for 5 minutes, then put a plate over the tin and flip over to turn out onto the plate. Peel off the baking paper and serve warm.

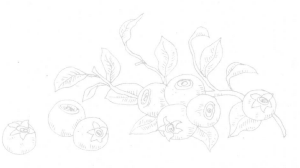

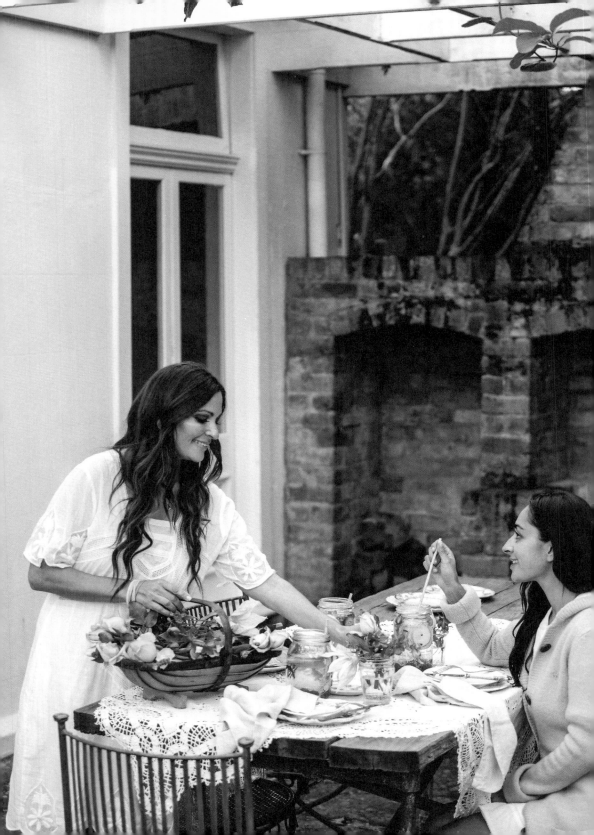

Recreating the lost art of mealtimes

When was the last time you sat down with friends or family to a meal? It baffles me hugely that as a culture we're so used to eating on the run that we've abandoned the beautiful, communal ritual of eating at the table.

Traditionally, the table was – and should still be – the focal point at mealtimes. These days, the TV, mobile phones and laptops have replaced it, and as a result, the powerful connection that occurs over a meal has been lost from many families and relationships.

If you asked someone from France about the differences between their culture and ours, you'd find that their answers would most certainly link back to food: the appreciation of food and the ritual of sitting down to eat at the table. In France, families, friends and co-workers will eat at the table for every meal. Even in kindergarten, children will sit down to lunch at a table, and are expected to use real glasses, ceramic plates and proper cutlery – no plastic.

In Australia and most of the West, we have a highly individualistic approach to eating, and as a result a lack of home hospitality. In France, there's no eating on the run, and there's a wonderful appreciation, joy and passion for food that I think should be at the heart of our meals.

Recreating the lost art of mealtimes will bring deeper satisfaction and respect for your food. It will strengthen your relationships, thus improving your health, as social interaction and connection with community have been shown to be one of the greatest enhancers of longevity.

Even if you're on your own during work hours, you can still take the time to incorporate a mealtime ritual into your day. Sit down at a table. Switch off the phone, put the paper aside and just be with your meal. Enjoy the simple act of eating again.

How to recreate the lost art of mealtimes:

- PRIORITISE MEALTIMES. Be home for breakfast and be home for dinner. If you're a parent, make it a core value that the family eats together. This will take work and scheduling, but it's worth it.

- TURN OFF THE TV. Eliminate distractions so that everyone eating is focused on their food and each other.

- WHEN AT HOME, ADD ATMOSPHERE. Freshly cut flowers from the garden in a vase, a new tablecloth, tea lights – whatever creates a vibe of hospitality to honour your mealtime.

- GIVE THANKS. Whatever you believe, be thankful for your meal. Say grace, a ritualistic prayer or quick affirmation of gratitude for the meal. This will bring focus to the meal, and making it a regular habit will give mealtimes greater meaning and enhance your family connections. If you're alone, it allows you to remain mindful of the blessing of food, framing it in a positive light.

- MAKE THE TABLE AN ENTICING PLACE TO BE (see page 315). Invest in long-lasting tableware or collect from op shops (charity or thrift shops) to create a culture of valuing mealtimes. When people approach a beautifully set table, they feel honoured and valued, and will be more likely to enjoy their time at the table.

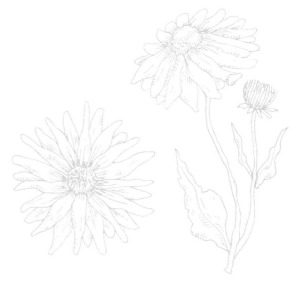

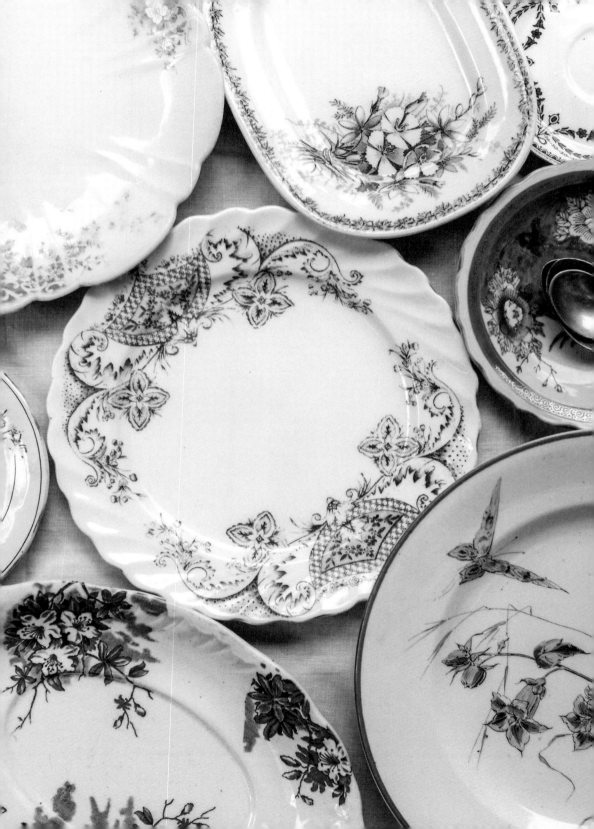

Setting the table

When I was growing up, setting the table was a big thing. Whether we were to be sitting cosy indoors in winter or taking a pew in the garden in summertime, I'd spread a fresh cloth on the table. Then, while Mum was busy getting the plates and cutlery together, not to mention the food, I'd be unearthing treasures to liven up the linen – gathering conkers, bark and leaves, and herbs from the garden, my mind busy and planning excitedly.

Even when I was only eight years old, I knew exactly what I wanted to do and how I wanted the table to look. Although we had only modest resources – no expensive flatware or bone china, and serving platters were scant – I used my imagination, and the beautiful elements gathered from the garden and repurposed for the table always enhanced our simple suppers. There was none of that old-fashioned formal stuffiness about our table, and it looked decidedly rustic!

One of my first table-setting jobs was to fold the cloth napkins into triangles. I usually kept away from fancy foldings, but occasionally a lopsided boat or bishop's hat would emerge. I'd try to remember to leave one spare for polishing the knives and forks, not always with success. The plates needed to be spaced evenly, with a napkin on top and then a drinking glass to the side. The cutlery was neatly arranged on either side of the plate, knife-edge facing the plate and standing straight, like a guard on his watch at Buckingham Palace.

This simple act was conducted with much anticipation for our nightly family dinner, which wouldn't always go exactly to plan, especially with two older sisters. Conversations were spontaneous and unpredictable, but it was nevertheless a chance to be together and let go of the complications of the day, or just chat about our daily happenings, or laugh, or mostly annoy each other. It was the reward at the end of the day, and although we grumbled during the meal, deep down we all loved it. It was us.

I decided that the fun part for me was all in the preparation and the anticipation of what was to come. My sisters pitched in sometimes, but their lack of enthusiasm meant they always

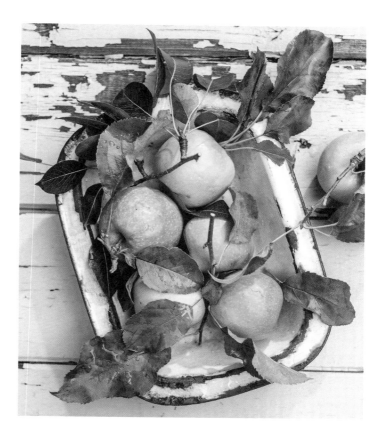

wanted to finish up quickly because they had something else that urgently needed to be done.

These are the simple lessons that are ingrained as a child and impossible to forget, but regrettably they've somehow slipped by the wayside for many of us in our modern culture. Back in the 1970s, people didn't make plans when it was time for dinner and no one called you on the phone. It's interesting to consider that although our smartphones have brought us closer to the rest of the world, they've catapulted us further away from our own families, and meaningful shared experiences and time spent together have become less frequent and less of a priority.

Being together at the family table is a chance to celebrate togetherness, whatever family model you have. Food is central to that, and should be embraced and enjoyed with the people we love. Keep reading for some of my favourite sit-down meals.

Mushroom and kale lasagne

{ *SERVES* 4 }

60 ml (2 fl oz/¼ cup) extra
   virgin olive oil

3 small zucchini (courgettes),
   cut into 5 mm (¼ inch) slices

½ brown onion, chopped

2 garlic cloves, crushed

300 g (10½ oz) mushrooms,
   sliced

350 g (12 oz/1 small bunch) kale,
   stems and spines removed,
   chopped

4 tomatoes, chopped

125 ml (4 fl oz/½ cup) tomato
   passata (puréed tomatoes)

2 tablespoons additive-free
   tomato paste (concentrated
   purée)

1½ teaspoons chopped fresh
   or dried herbs (e.g. oregano,
   sage, basil and thyme)

freshly ground black pepper,
   to taste

200 g (7 oz/¾ cup) plain
   sheep's yoghurt or plain
   Greek yoghurt

2 tablespoons nutritional yeast
   flakes or 150 g (5½ oz/
   1½ cups) grated cheddar
   cheese

Preheat the oven to 200°C (400°F).

Heat 2 tablespoons of the olive oil in a large frying pan over medium–high heat and fry the zucchini on both sides until golden. Remove from the pan and set aside.

In the same frying pan, heat the remaining oil then brown the onion and garlic. Add the mushrooms and kale, cook until tender, then add the tomatoes, tomato passata, tomato paste and herbs. Reduce the heat to low and simmer for 15 minutes. Season with pepper.

Assemble the lasagne by layering the ingredients in a baking dish: Start with half of the mushroom and tomato mixture, followed by half the zucchini and then half of the yoghurt. Repeat the layers then sprinkle with nutritional yeast and bake for 25 minutes.

Stand for 10 minutes before serving.

Whole baked salmon with parsley and walnuts

{ *SERVES 6–8* }

3–4 kg (6 lb 12 oz–8 lb 13 oz) fresh whole salmon, scaled and gutted

60 ml (2 fl oz/¼ cup) extra virgin olive oil, plus extra for drizzling

3 lemons, 1 halved, 2 sliced

sea salt and freshly ground black pepper, to taste

handful flat-leaf (Italian) parsley, chopped

115 g (4 oz/1 cup) walnuts, chopped

Preheat the oven to 180°C (350°F).

Wash the salmon and pat it dry with paper towel inside and out. Lay a sheet of foil on a large baking tray. Lay the fish in the centre of the tray (or diagonally if too large), drizzle over the olive oil and squeeze over the juice from one lemon half. Place lemon slices inside the salmon and some more on top. Season well with salt and pepper. Seal the foil to make a loose parcel.

Bake for 30 minutes or until the salmon is cooked through — check by inserting a skewer or sharp knife into the thickest part of the fish, just behind the head. About halfway through cooking, open the parcel, add the parsley and walnuts, then reseal. When the fish is cooked, remove the foil, squeeze over the juice from the remaining lemon half and drizzle over extra olive oil.

Eat straight away or refrigerate overnight. Use any left-over salmon to whip up my Asparagus, Mushroom and Salmon Frittata (page 230) for lunch!

Pulled pork with kaleslaw

{ *SERVES 6* }

Pulled pork is one of the most satisfying comfort foods. To really max out on flavour and tenderness, it's important to find a good butcher who is passionate about providing organic free-range pork. They should know the farmer and be aware of the farming practices used. This is a dish to wow dinner guests and really pour your love and care into preparing. In fact, love is the key ingredient!

1 large free-range pork shoulder, bone removed

2 tablespoons olive oil

1½ teaspoons sea salt

250 ml (9 fl oz/1 cup) apple cider vinegar, plus extra as needed

Kaleslaw with Creamy Sesame Dressing (page 123), to serve

Dry rub

2 garlic cloves

1 dried chilli or 2 teaspoons chilli flakes

2 tablespoons fennel seeds

2 tablespoons smoked paprika

1 tablespoon black peppercorns

1 teaspoon coriander seeds

1 teaspoon cumin seeds

90 g (3¼ oz/¼ cup) rice malt syrup

Preheat the oven to 220°C (425°F).

Score the pork skin about 1 cm (½ inch) deep with a sharp knife. Drizzle over half the olive oil and sprinkle over the salt.

To make the dry rub, use a mortar and pestle to pound together all the ingredients except the rice malt syrup to release their flavours. Mix with the rice malt syrup in a small bowl.

Heat the remaining olive oil in a flameproof casserole dish over medium heat on the stovetop and brown the pork on both sides. Remove from the heat and allow to cool then work the dry rub into the pork, ensuring you push it into all the creases. Drain the excess fat from the dish and pour the vinegar over the pork. Cover and transfer to the oven for 20 minutes, then reduce the heat to 140°C (275°F) and roast for 4 hours, topping up with apple cider vinegar periodically if needed, until the meat is tender and pulls apart easily. Remove from the oven then shred the pork using two forks.

Serve the pulled pork with the crackling and with kaleslaw with creamy sesame dressing.

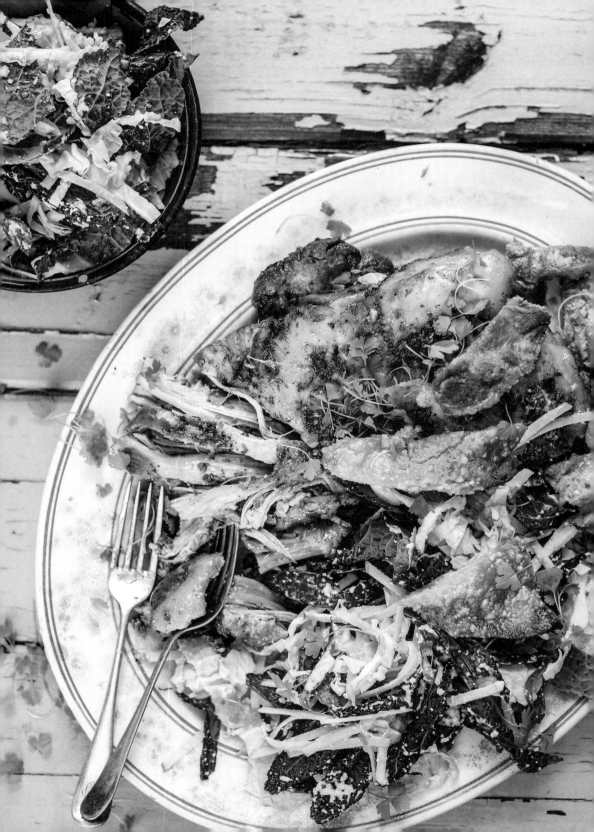

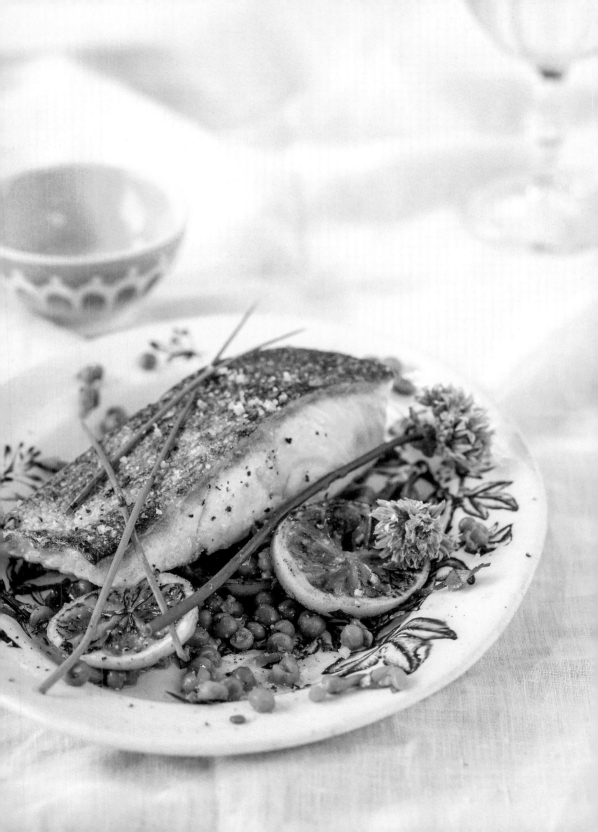

Crispy salmon with saffron aioli and smashed green peas

{ *SERVES* 4 }

4 salmon fillets, skin on

sea salt, for rubbing

2 tablespoons olive oil

1 lemon, sliced and roasted, to serve (optional)

chives and edible flowers, to serve (optional)

Saffron aioli

2 garlic cloves, crushed

2 teaspoons lemon juice

1/2 teaspoon sea salt

2 egg yolks

1 tablespoon dijon mustard

pinch of saffron threads, soaked in a little lemon juice

375 ml (13 fl oz/1½ cups) extra virgin olive oil

sea salt and freshly ground black pepper, to taste

Smashed peas

200 g (7 oz) frozen peas

50 ml (1¾ fl oz) vegetable stock or filtered water

pinch of sea salt

30 g (1 oz) butter

juice of 1 lemon

freshly ground black pepper, to taste

1 tablespoon olive oil

2 tablespoons chopped flat-leaf (Italian) parsley

handful mint leaves

1 tablespoon snipped chives

To make the saffron aioli, whiz the garlic, lemon juice, salt, egg yolks and mustard in a food processor. Add the saffron and process again. With the motor still running, very slowly drizzle in the olive oil. The mixture will emulsify to a mayonnaise-like consistency. Season to taste.

To make the smashed peas, put the peas and stock in a medium saucepan, season with salt and cook over medium–high heat, stirring occasionally, until the peas are tender. Remove from the heat, strain and stir in the butter. Gently mash the peas with a fork, then stir in the lemon juice and black pepper. Mix in the olive oil a little at a time, until the peas have the desired consistency. Fold in the herbs.

Pat the salmon dry with paper towel and rub salt into the skin. Heat a large frying pan over medium–high heat, then add the olive oil and heat until the oil shimmers. Place the salmon fillets in the pan, skin side down, and press on them with a spatula to ensure all of the skin is in contact with the pan. Cook for 4–5 minutes, until the skin is crispy and the salmon is still pink inside. Turn over with a spatula, turn off the heat and let the fish sit in the pan for no more than 1 minute.

Divide the smashed peas between four serving plates and top with the salmon and the roasted lemon slices, if using. Garnish with chives and edible flowers, if using, and serve with the aioli on the side.

Butterflied roast chicken with tarator sauce and herb and pistachio salad

{ *SERVES* 4 }

1 chicken

sea salt and freshly ground
black pepper, to taste

2 tablespoons olive oil

juice of 2 lemons

1 teaspoon dried oregano

6 garlic cloves, peeled

a few thyme sprigs

seeds of 1 pomegranate (optional)

Tarator sauce

200 g (7 oz/³/₄ cup) full-fat
plain yoghurt

135 g (4³/₄ oz/¹/₂ cup) tahini

1 teaspoon grated lemon zest

60 ml (2 fl oz/¹/₄ cup) lemon juice

2 teaspoons ground cumin

1 teaspoon sumac or extra
lemon zest

1 garlic clove, peeled

1 tablespoon chopped parsley

125 ml (4 fl oz/¹/₂ cup) filtered
water

Herb and pistachio salad

2 tablespoons extra virgin olive oil

2 tablespoons lemon juice

sea salt and freshly ground
black pepper, to taste

large handful coriander
(cilantro) leaves

large handful mint leaves

35 g (1¹/₄ oz/1 tightly packed
cup) rocket (arugula)

1 red onion

90 g (3¹/₄ oz/²/₃ cup) pistachio
nut kernels

Preheat the oven to 200°C (400°F).

Lay the chicken on a clean work surface, cut along the backbone using kitchen shears, then butterfly the bird by opening out the legs and spreading the body flat, skin side up. Flatten more by pressing on the breastbone with your hands. You can ask your butcher to do the butterflying for you. Pat the chicken dry with paper towel and move to a roasting tin.

Season the bird generously with salt and pepper. Drizzle over the olive oil and lemon juice, scatter over the oregano and tuck the garlic and thyme into the folds. Bake for 1 hour 20 minutes, or until the chicken is golden brown and cooked through.

Meanwhile, make the tarator sauce. In a mini-blender, whiz the yoghurt, tahini, lemon zest and juice, cumin, sumac, garlic and parsley, then add enough of the water to make a creamy sauce.

Prepare the salad by whisking the olive oil, lemon juice, salt and pepper in a medium bowl. Chop the coriander and mint, tear the rocket, and finely chop the onion. Add the herbs, rocket and onion to the dressing with the pistachio nuts. Toss well.

To serve, lay the chicken on a platter and drizzle over the tarator sauce or serve on the side. Add the salad around the chicken and scatter over the pomegranate seeds, if using.

Seared beef with mushrooms and sage nut butter sauce on watercress salad

{ SERVES 2 }

I love to express my creativity in the kitchen, but at heart I'm very content with a protein and salad dinner. My only requirements are meat of the best quality, and vegies grown with love and organic principles. This really amps up the flavour.

2 teaspoons sesame oil

2 rib-eye steaks

sea salt and freshly ground black pepper, to taste

2 tablespoons sesame seeds

40 g (1½ oz) or 2 tablespoons butter olive oil

180 g (6¼ oz/2 cups) sliced mushrooms

Sage nut butter sauce

60 g (2¼ oz/¼ cup) nut butter

60 ml (2 fl oz/¼ cup) coconut milk

large handful sage leaves

sea salt and freshly ground black pepper, to taste

Watercress salad

120 g (4¼ oz/4 cups) watercress

1 orange, peeled and cut into segments or unpeeled and sliced

1 teaspoon grated orange zest

1 tablespoon orange juice (see tip)

2 tablespoons olive oil

1 tablespoon rice malt syrup or stevia to taste (optional)

To make the sage nut butter sauce, gently melt the nut butter and coconut milk in a small saucepan over low heat and add the sage. Cook very gently for 5–8 minutes, taking care not to let it boil. Season with salt and pepper.

To make the watercress salad, combine the watercress and the orange segments in a medium bowl. Whisk the remaining ingredients in a small bowl, pour over the salad and toss.

Rub the sesame oil all over the steaks, season with salt and pepper and sprinkle with sesame seeds, pressing down to ensure they stick. Heat half the butter in a large frying pan over medium–high heat. Sauté the mushrooms for about 8 minutes, until browned, and season with salt and pepper. Transfer to a plate.

Heat the remaining butter in the same frying pan over medium–high heat, then cook the steaks to your liking. Transfer the steaks to a cutting board and slice on the diagonal using a sharp knife.

Share the salad between two plates. Top with steak slices and mushrooms, and serve with the sage nut butter sauce on the side.

Note: For a photo of this dish, see pages 332–33.

Slow-cooked braised lamb with roasted carrots

{ *SERVES* 4-6 }

I honestly don't know what I'd do without my slow-cooker. I use it to make broths; to cook beans, stews and soups; and – my favourite – for the long, slow cooking of meats. I've written this recipe for the oven, as not everyone has a slow-cooker, but if you do, feel free to use that and cook on low for 6 to 8 hours. (For more flavour, you can seal the lamb in a pan over a medium heat with a tablespoon of olive oil prior.) This lamb shoulder becomes so soft and buttery, flaking and sliding away from itself. It's truly divine, and the most scrumptious meal to come home to after a long day at work.

1 × 2 kg (4 lb 8 oz) leg of lamb or lamb shoulder

4 garlic cloves, sliced

6 anchovy fillets, cut in half

sea salt and freshly ground black pepper, to taste

250 ml (9 fl oz/1 cup) almond milk or water

1 cinnamon stick

1 fennel bulb, quartered

bunch baby carrots

oregano leaves, to serve

Marinade

1 tablespoon cumin seeds, toasted and lightly crushed

1 tablespoon fennel seeds

1 tablespoon ground cinnamon

90 g (3¼ oz/¼ cup) rice malt syrup

2 tablespoons olive oil

grated zest and juice of 1 lemon

Preheat the oven to 175°C (345°F).

Using a small knife, make incisions all over the meat and insert the garlic and anchovies.

Mix together the marinade ingredients to form a thick paste, then rub all over the lamb using your hands.

Sit the lamb in a roasting tin or casserole dish. Season with salt and pepper, pour over the almond milk and add the cinnamon stick. Cover with foil and roast for 2½–3 hours, basting regularly during cooking. Add the vegetables for the final 30–60 minutes, or roast separately.

Remove from the oven, remove the foil, cover with a tea towel (dish towel) and allow to rest for about 10 minutes. Carve the meat and serve with the fennel, carrots and cooking juices, topped with the oregano.

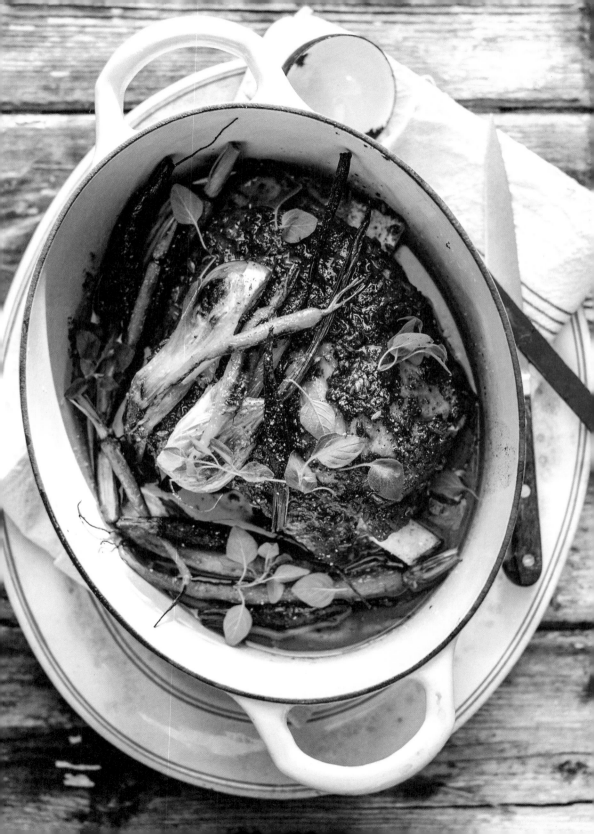

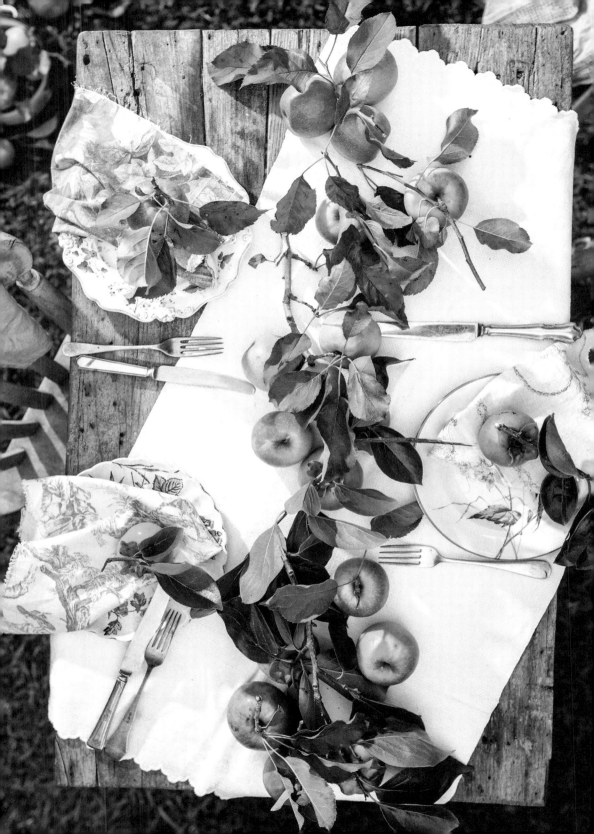

Simple tablescapes

Whether it's a special occasion or an everyday meal, here are some uncomplicated and inexpensive ways to upcycle discarded objects and decorate your table, elevating your food and turning gatherings into inviting communal feasts.

Follow these steps to create your simple settings:

1   First, choose a theme, so that you can create a beautiful cohesive arrangement. You can base it on any particular approach you like: garden style with bits and bobs from the garden; ocean style with shells and coral you picked up on your last visit to the beach; clean style with simple elements and colour scheme; or bohemian with a mixture of different patterns and textures. Find a feel you like or experiment as you go along.

2   Decide on a base. You could choose a plain white table cloth or a boldly coloured one, or even ditch the cloth altogether and use a runner made with a piece of fabric – even inexpensive brown paper looks fantastic as a runner. A piece of old wood can double as a fun runner, too.

3   Find plates you like. I like to shop at second-hand stores for seasonal and quirky plates with a vintage feel.

4   Now for the fun part; it's time for decorating! Try the ideas on the following pages and let your creative juices flow. Whether you're preparing a dinner for one, a romantic supper for lovebirds, a family gathering or special occasion, or a simple picnic lunch with friends – on a rug, carpet or even the patio – you'll find extra inspiration on pages 330–37.

FUSS-FREE TABLE-SCAPES

Try these tips:

- Mix and match. Not everything needs to be matchy-matchy. Use contrasting textures, patterns and colours. If you don't have a complete set of plates, for example, mix them up and think about using the overall setting to bring them together.

- Let food provide the colours on the table – citrus fruits and pumpkins always look gorgeous, and you can give them to your gathering to take home to enjoy later. You can also use fruit such as oranges and pomegranates as place markers.

- Use cinnamon sticks, lavender or rosemary to create a beautiful aroma at the table.

- Use vintage tea towels (dish towels), which can be found in op shops very cheaply, for napkins. Placemats can be made from small square pillowcases or cushion covers. Omit napkin rings and instead use ribbon or natural twine tied in a bow with a sprig of rosemary or, say, rhubarb stalks and radishes (see page 319). Keep it simple.

- For a larger gathering, place the cutlery in a wooden box or rustic second-hand container or tin.

- If you're planning a breakfast, serve boiled eggs in their shells and put them back in their cartons, or fill egg cartons with flowers and leaves as table decorations. You can also plant herbs in used eggshells and put them back in the carton as a decoration.

- Upcycle your flea market finds, unearth treasures in junk shops, and use different old tins and cans with a mixture of flowers to create a boho look. Save your spice jars and glass jars of varying shapes and sizes, and cluster them together. Jars and pots can also be used to bring out fresh home-made condiments.

- For outdoor gatherings and picnics, use flower pots as garden-inspired utensil holders. Tissue-paper pompoms are fun and easy to make too. Value the environment and share your passion for it by repurposing.

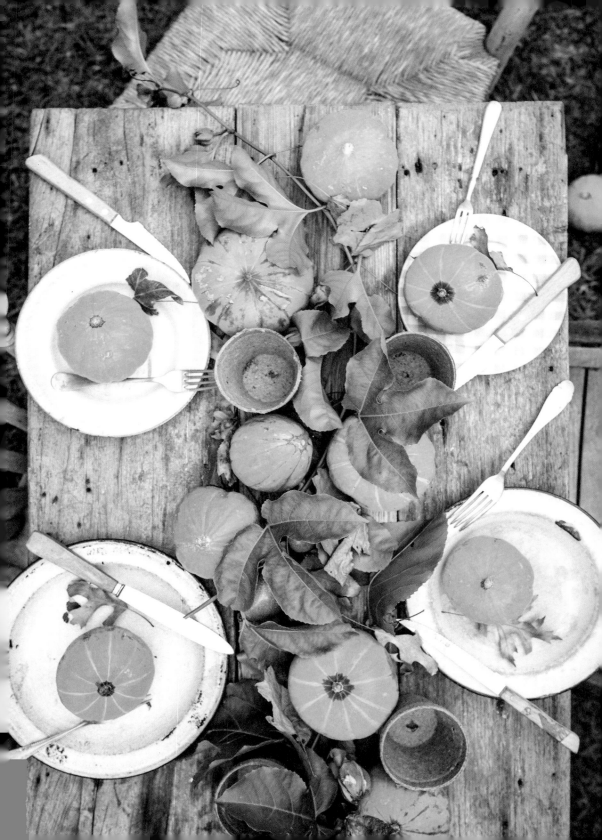

BEAUTY IN THE EVERYDAY

Your decorating ideas needn't be fancy to be really effective. For Christmas last year I used decorating magazines as placemats. They were a big talking point and everyone wanted to take them home afterwards. If you're planning a gathering, make menu cards with brown paper. You can also use it to name your ingredients or even wrap cutlery or gift-wrap fresh herbs. Or put your cutlery in brown paper bags and tie the tops with twine or ribbon, or just fold them over.

Real plants and foliage offer free table décor, and you can give them to your friends to take home as a simple and sweet gift. Twigs, colourful leaves, branches and plants such as jasmine look beautiful as a centrepiece or runner. Cut sprigs and weave them across the table. It's fun being a forager! Bring some sparkle to the room by hanging pressed autumn leaves on fishing line from the dining room or kitchen window.

Take upcycling to the max and make merry by re-using jars to create stunning snow globes. Glue down small objects or ornaments from around the house, and use desiccated coconut as snow.

Turn your next trip to the beach into a treasure hunt. It's amazing what you can find. Pick up shells, coral, driftwood and feathers, and use them to decorate your table. All you need is a bit of creativity.

If you gear your table towards simplicity, naturalness and eco-consciousness, it can look authentic and needn't cost you an arm and a leg.

Ready for a supercharged Christmas menu? Turn the page.

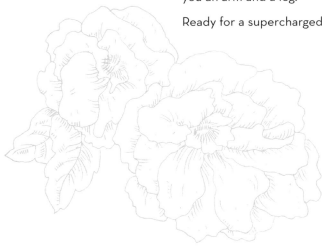

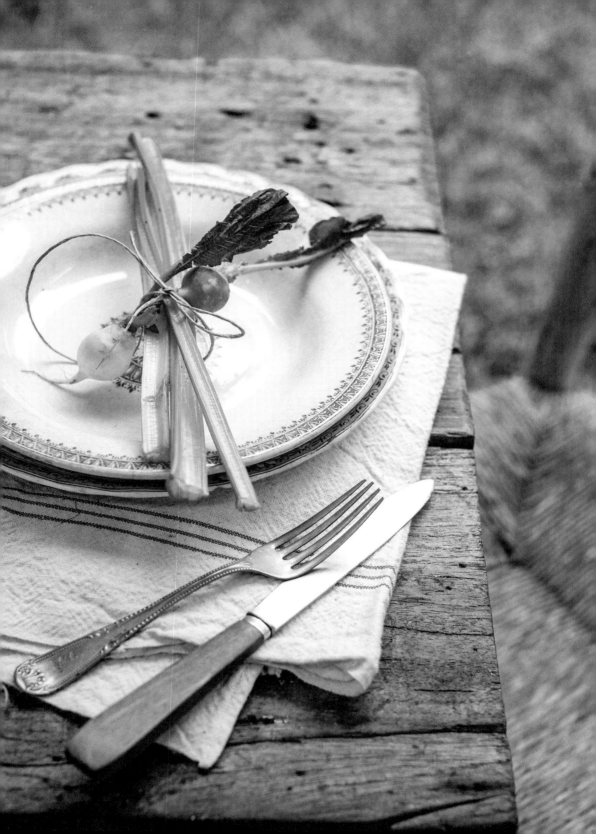

Coconut egg nog

{ *SERVES 6* }

250 ml (9 fl oz/1 cup) coconut
 cream

750 ml (26 fl oz/3 cups) coconut
 milk

3 cinnamon sticks

1 teaspoon ground cinnamon,
 plus extra to serve

1 teaspoon freshly grated
 nutmeg, plus extra to serve

1 teaspoon vanilla powder

5 egg yolks

Combine all the ingredients except the egg
yolks in a medium saucepan, stir gently until
combined, then slowly bring to the boil over
medium-low heat. Remove from the heat and
set aside to steep for 3-4 minutes.

Whiz the egg yolks in a blender on high until
frothy. Add the coconut milk mixture, then
whiz for a couple more seconds.

Serve warm or chilled, sprinkled with extra
cinnamon and nutmeg.

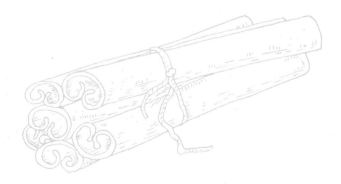

Pistachio minted cranberry quinoa

{ *SERVES* 4 }

olive oil, for frying (optional)

300 g (10½ oz/1½ cups) white quinoa, thoroughly rinsed and drained

500 ml (17 fl oz/2 cups) chicken stock

½ teaspoon sea salt (optional), plus extra to serve

105 g (3¾ oz/²/₃ cup) cranberries

90 g (3¼ oz/²/₃ cup) pistachio nut kernels

2 tablespoons lemon oil (see note page 48)

1 tablespoon apple cider vinegar

1 tablespoon lemon juice

freshly ground black pepper, to taste

Heat a drizzle of olive oil, if using, in a large saucepan over medium–high heat, and add the quinoa. Cook, stirring, for about 1 minute to let the rinsing water evaporate and toast the quinoa. (This brings out the earthy flavour.) Stir in the chicken stock and salt, if using, then bring to a rolling boil. Reduce the heat to low and simmer, covered, for 12–15 minutes, until the quinoa is cooked. Remove from the heat and stand, covered, in the saucepan for 5 minutes.

Fluff the quinoa gently with a fork and transfer to a large bowl. Add the remaining ingredients, and mix well. Adjust the seasoning and serve.

Caramelised baked sweet potatoes

{ *SERVES* 10–12 }

Bake these with the turkey (page 322) if you have room!

2 teaspoons coconut sugar

¼ teaspoon freshly grated nutmeg

1 teaspoon sea salt

6 sweet potatoes, peeled and cut into long batons

2 tablespoons coconut oil, melted

Preheat the oven to 180°C (350°F). In a large bowl, mix the coconut sugar, nutmeg and salt. Add the sweet potato and coconut oil, and toss until the sweet potato is well coated.

Spread out the sweet potato on a baking tray. Bake for about 1 hour, until deep golden brown all over, turning halfway through.

Roasted whole turkey

{ SERVES 10–12 }

You can serve this with my Easy-peasy Minted Peas with Goat's Cheese and Bacon (page 96).

1 × 6 kg (13 lb 4 oz) turkey, giblets removed

large handful flat-leaf (Italian) parsley

sea salt and freshly ground black pepper

170 g (6 oz) butter, softened

grated zest and juice of 1 lemon

large handful thyme

small handful sage

3 bay leaves (optional)

2 brown onions, peeled and halved

2 leeks, pale part only, halved lengthways

4 baby carrots, halved

2 celery stalks, halved lengthways

2 garlic bulbs

1 litre (35 fl oz/4 cups) chicken stock

Preheat the oven to 210°C (410°F).

Pat the turkey dry with paper towel. Place the parsley in the cavity. Season the turkey with salt and pepper, and place in a large roasting tin. Spread the butter all over the bird. Drizzle over the lemon juice, sprinkle over the zest, and tuck the remaining herbs under the bird.

Arrange the onion, leek, carrot, celery and whole garlic bulbs around the turkey, then pour in the stock. Cover the tin with foil and roast for 45 minutes, then reduce the oven temperature to 170°C (325°F) and roast for a further 3–4 hours. About 10 minutes before the end of cooking, remove the foil, increase the oven temperature to 200°C (400°F) and roast until the turkey skin is golden brown and crisp, and the juices from the thickest part of the leg run clear.

Remove from the oven and set aside to rest for at least 15 minutes before carving.

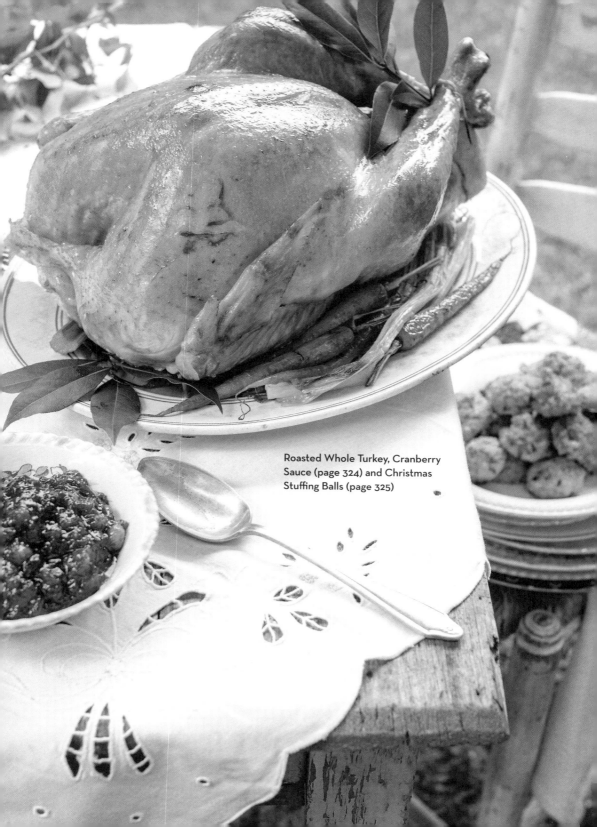

Roasted Whole Turkey, Cranberry Sauce (page 324) and Christmas Stuffing Balls (page 325)

Cranberry sauce

{ *MAKES ABOUT 500 ML [17 FL OZ/2 CUPS]* }

310 g (11 oz/2½ cups) fresh
  cranberries, rinsed and
  drained, or frozen cranberries

180 g (6¼ oz/½ cup) rice malt
  syrup, plus extra as needed

125 ml (4 fl oz/½ cup) filtered
  water

grated zest of 1 orange

1 tablespoon apple cider
  vinegar

½ teaspoon ground cinnamon

Combine all the ingredients in a small
saucepan and bring to a gentle boil over
medium heat. Reduce the heat to medium–low
and simmer, stirring, for about 10 minutes, until
the mixture thickens.

Taste for sweetness, add more rice malt syrup
if necessary, then cool and seal in a sterilised
jar until ready to use.

Christmas stuffing balls

{ *MAKES* 12 }

These can be made the day before and warmed in the oven while the turkey rests – 10 minutes at 150°C (300°C) should do the trick.

2 tablespoons extra virgin olive oil

1 large brown onion, finely chopped

2 garlic cloves, crushed

2 celery stalks, finely chopped

500 g (1 lb 2 oz) minced (ground) pork

1 tablespoon dried mixed herbs (e.g. sage, rosemary, thyme)

2 tablespoons chopped parsley, plus extra to serve

1 tablespoon lemon zest

110 g (3¾ oz/½ cup) cooked quinoa or 95 g (3¼ oz/½ cup) cooked brown rice

115 g (4 oz/¾ cup) pine nuts or crushed nuts

100 g (3½ oz/1 cup) almond meal

2 eggs, lightly beaten

fine sea salt and freshly ground black pepper, to taste

Preheat the oven to 190°C (375°F) and grease a baking tray.

Heat the olive oil in a medium saucepan over medium heat, then sauté the onion, garlic and celery for 3–4 minutes, until the onion is translucent. Add the pork, mixed herbs, parsley and lemon zest, then cook until the pork is no longer pink. Add the quinoa and allow to cool.

Once cool, add the remaining ingredients and mix well.

Roll 60 g (2¼ oz/¼ cup) portions of the mixture into balls, sit them on the prepared baking tray, then bake for 30 minutes, or until golden brown and crispy.

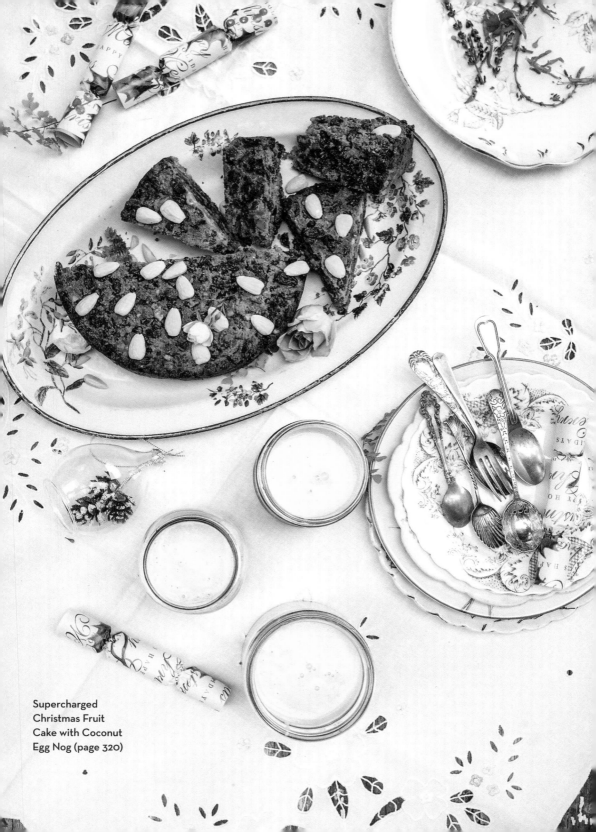

Supercharged
Christmas Fruit
Cake with Coconut
Egg Nog (page 320)

Supercharged Christmas fruit cake

{ *MAKES ONE 22 CM [8½ INCH] CAKE* }

200 g (7 oz/2 cups) almond meal

50 g (1¾ oz) walnuts, chopped

650 g (1 lb 7 oz) mixed dried fruit (e.g. currants, cranberries, blueberries, raisins, figs, apricots, sultanas, cherries, dates)

½ teaspoon ground cinnamon

½ teaspoon allspice

¼ teaspoon ground ginger

¼ teaspoon freshly grated nutmeg

1 teaspoon gluten-free baking powder

½ teaspoon bicarbonate of soda (baking soda)

1 teaspoon vanilla powder or alcohol-free vanilla extract

pinch of sea salt

1 tablespoon grated lemon zest

60 ml (2 fl oz/¼ cup) lemon juice

80 ml (2½ fl oz/⅓ cup) coconut milk

80 ml (2½ fl oz/⅓ cup) walnut oil, almond oil or light olive oil

3 eggs, lightly beaten

80 g (2¾ oz/½ cup) blanched almonds, to decorate

Preheat the oven to 160°C (315°F). Grease a 22 cm (8½ inch) round cake tin and line it with baking paper.

In a large bowl, combine the almond meal, walnuts, dried fruit, spices, baking powder, bicarbonate of soda, vanilla powder, salt and lemon zest.

In a separate large bowl whisk together the lemon juice, coconut milk, walnut oil and eggs. Add the dry ingredients to the wet and fold through. Spoon the mixture into the prepared tin, then press down using your hands so that it is compact and tightly packed. Smooth the top with the back of a spoon if necessary.

Bake for 1 hour on the middle shelf of the oven. Remove the cake, press the blanched almonds into the top, then return to the oven for 30 minutes, or until a skewer inserted in the centre comes out clean.

Cool completely in the tin, then remove carefully. It will keep in an airtight container in the fridge for up to 1 month.

Mango cheesecake

{ MAKES ONE 20 CM [8 INCH] CAKE }

Looking for the perfect Aussie Christmas dessert? Yes, I know, a cheese-less cheesecake ... but sometimes you just have to trust me! I think I can even say that I like this more than regular cheesecake. Don't be the friend who brings the unpalatable raw dessert to your Christmas lunch party. Bring this instead!

handful mixed berries, to serve

Base

250 g (9 oz) raw cashews, soaked in filtered water for 2 hours

100 g (3½ oz/1½ cups) shredded coconut

pinch of sea salt

60 ml (2 fl oz/¼ cup) lemon juice

2 tablespoons melted coconut butter

Filling

250 g (9 oz) cashews, soaked in filtered water for 2 hours, drained

120 g (4¼ oz/½ cup) coconut butter

3 fresh or frozen mangoes, diced

80 ml (2½ fl oz/⅓ cup) lemon juice

1 teaspoon vanilla extract

2 tablespoons rice malt syrup

80 ml (2½ fl oz/⅓ cup) coconut milk

Grease a 20 cm (8 inch) spring-form cake tin and line the bottom with baking paper.

To make the base, drain the soaked cashews, then combine the nuts and coconut in blender or food processor and chop finely. Turn out into a medium bowl.

Stir in the remaining ingredients, adding a little filtered water if necessary to help the mixture hold together.

Push the nut mixture into the prepared tin and set aside in the freezer while you make the filling.

To make the filling, whiz all the ingredients in a blender or food processor until smooth.

Remove the base from the freezer and spoon in the filling, smoothing the top with a spatula.

Return the cake to the freezer (or put it in the fridge) until set.

Top with the mixed berries and serve.

Mango sorbet

{ *SERVES* 2–3 }

If you're short of time, make this instead of the cheesecake – or strike while the mangoes are perfect and make both!

945 g (2 lb/3 cups) frozen mango chunks

125 ml (4 fl oz/½ cup) unsweetened pineapple juice, plus extra as needed

60 ml (2 fl oz/¼ cup) coconut milk or almond milk

Whiz all the ingredients in a high-speed blender until smooth, adding a little liquid if necessary. Serve immediately.

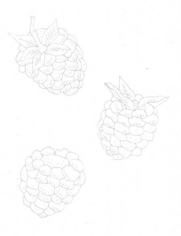

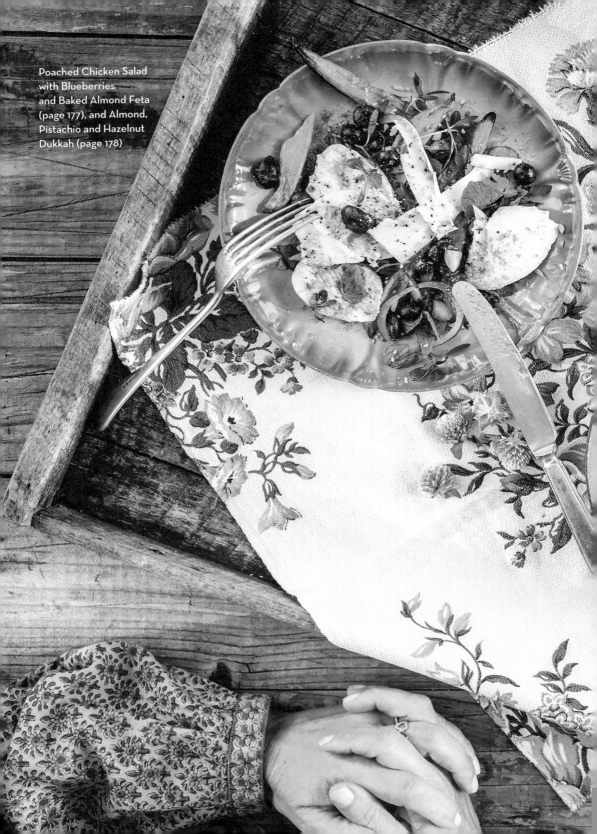

Poached Chicken Salad
with Blueberries
and Baked Almond Feta
(page 177), and Almond,
Pistachio and Hazelnut
Dukkah (page 178)

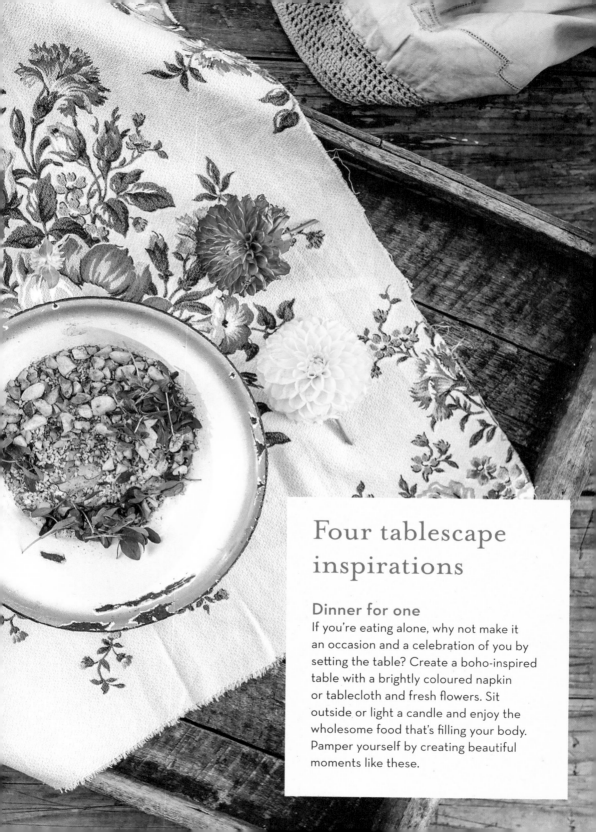

Four tablescape inspirations

Dinner for one
If you're eating alone, why not make it an occasion and a celebration of you by setting the table? Create a boho-inspired table with a brightly coloured napkin or tablecloth and fresh flowers. Sit outside or light a candle and enjoy the wholesome food that's filling your body. Pamper yourself by creating beautiful moments like these.

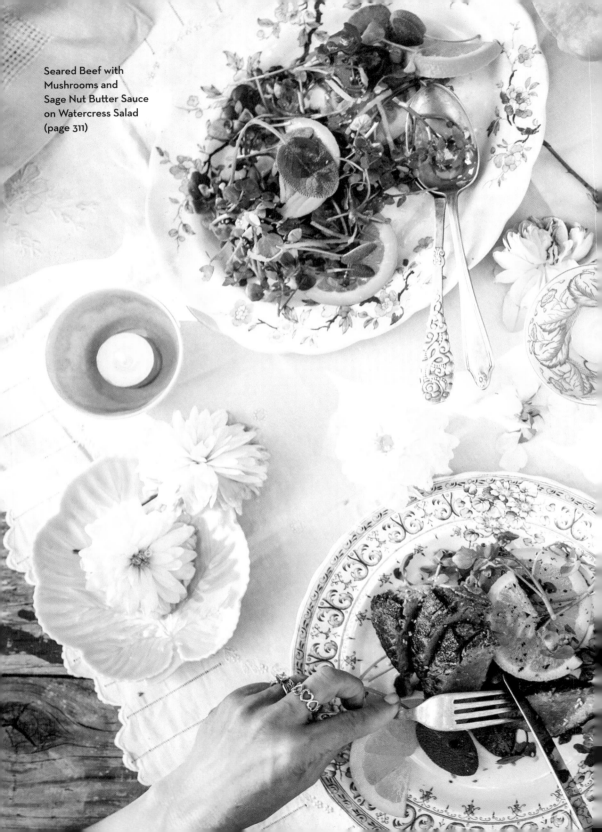

Seared Beef with
Mushrooms and
Sage Nut Butter Sauce
on Watercress Salad
(page 311)

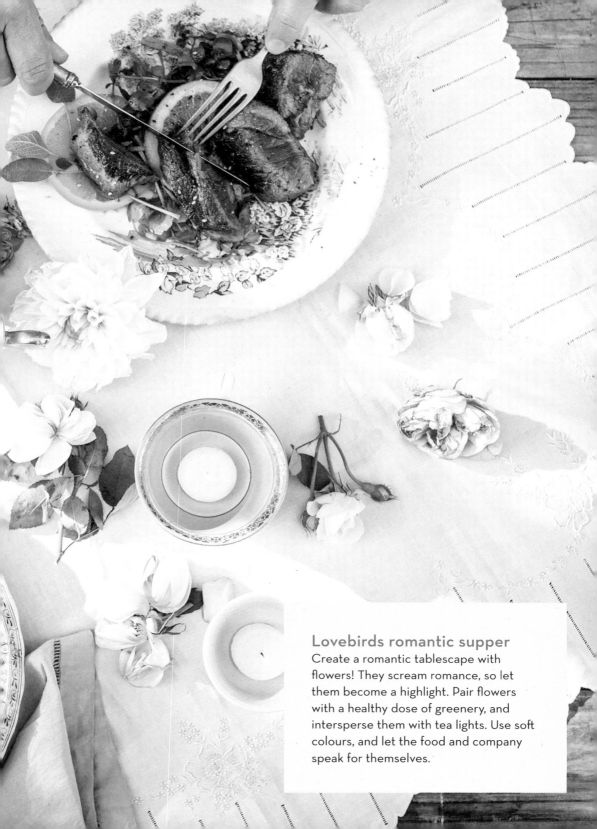

Lovebirds romantic supper

Create a romantic tablescape with flowers! They scream romance, so let them become a highlight. Pair flowers with a healthy dose of greenery, and intersperse them with tea lights. Use soft colours, and let the food and company speak for themselves.

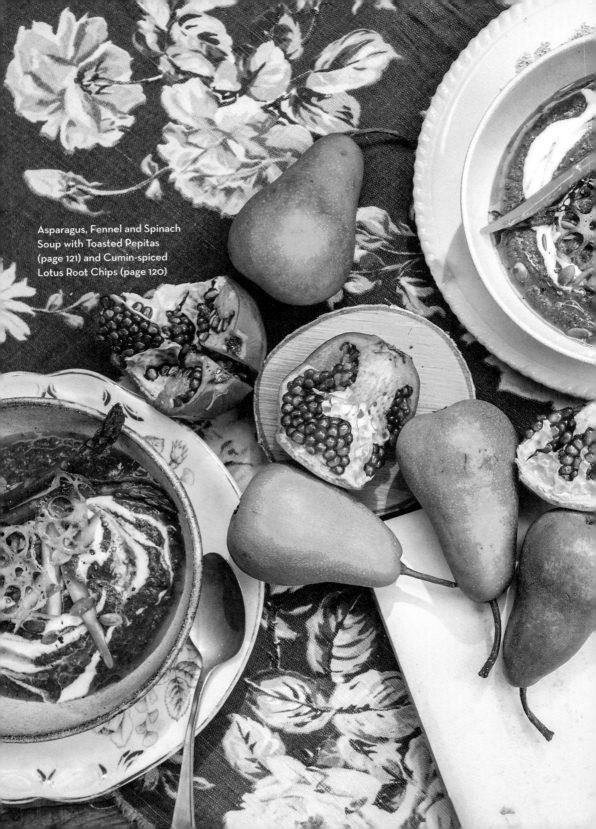

Asparagus, Fennel and Spinach
Soup with Toasted Pepitas
(page 121) and Cumin-spiced
Lotus Root Chips (page 120)

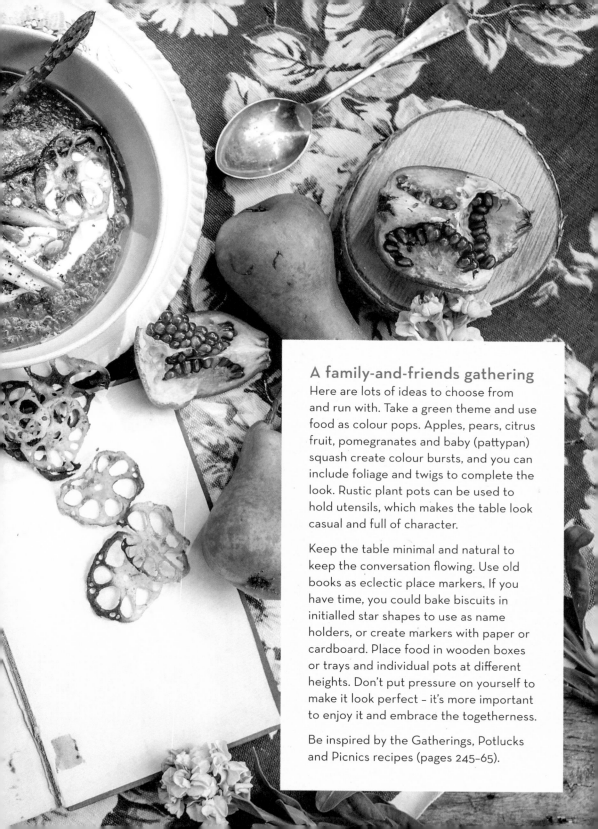

A family-and-friends gathering

Here are lots of ideas to choose from and run with. Take a green theme and use food as colour pops. Apples, pears, citrus fruit, pomegranates and baby (pattypan) squash create colour bursts, and you can include foliage and twigs to complete the look. Rustic plant pots can be used to hold utensils, which makes the table look casual and full of character.

Keep the table minimal and natural to keep the conversation flowing. Use old books as eclectic place markers. If you have time, you could bake biscuits in initialled star shapes to use as name holders, or create markers with paper or cardboard. Place food in wooden boxes or trays and individual pots at different heights. Don't put pressure on yourself to make it look perfect – it's more important to enjoy it and embrace the togetherness.

Be inspired by the Gatherings, Potlucks and Picnics recipes (pages 245–65).

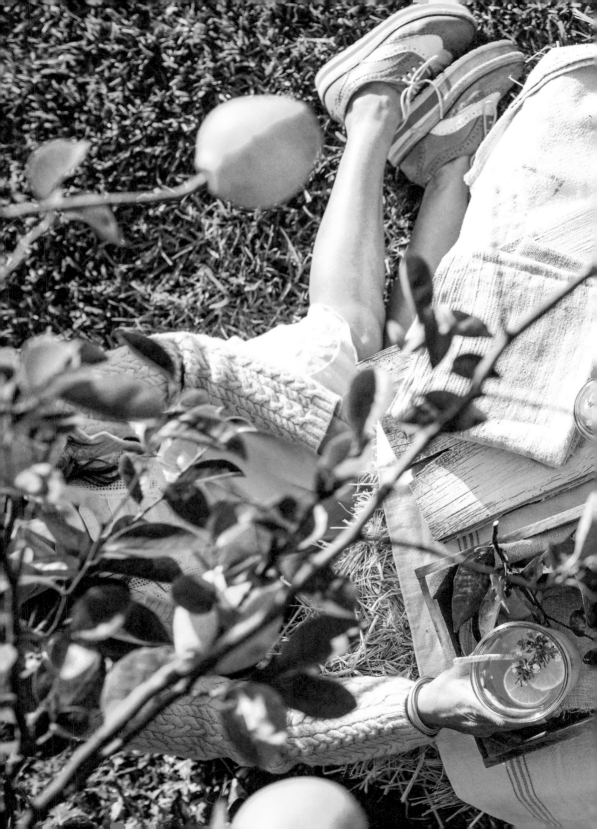

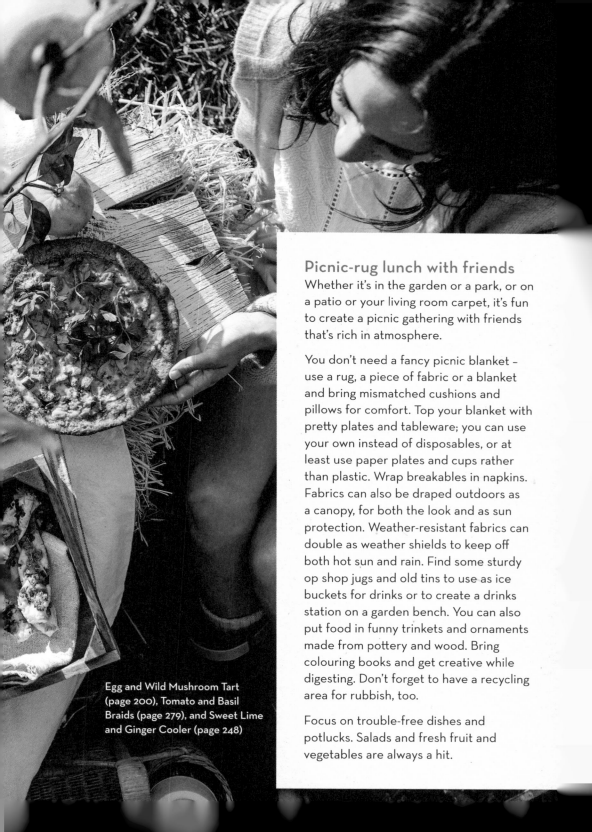

Picnic-rug lunch with friends

Whether it's in the garden or a park, or on a patio or your living room carpet, it's fun to create a picnic gathering with friends that's rich in atmosphere.

You don't need a fancy picnic blanket – use a rug, a piece of fabric or a blanket and bring mismatched cushions and pillows for comfort. Top your blanket with pretty plates and tableware; you can use your own instead of disposables, or at least use paper plates and cups rather than plastic. Wrap breakables in napkins. Fabrics can also be draped outdoors as a canopy, for both the look and as sun protection. Weather-resistant fabrics can double as weather shields to keep off both hot sun and rain. Find some sturdy op shop jugs and old tins to use as ice buckets for drinks or to create a drinks station on a garden bench. You can also put food in funny trinkets and ornaments made from pottery and wood. Bring colouring books and get creative while digesting. Don't forget to have a recycling area for rubbish, too.

Focus on trouble-free dishes and potlucks. Salads and fresh fruit and vegetables are always a hit.

Egg and Wild Mushroom Tart (page 200), Tomato and Basil Braids (page 279), and Sweet Lime and Ginger Cooler (page 248)

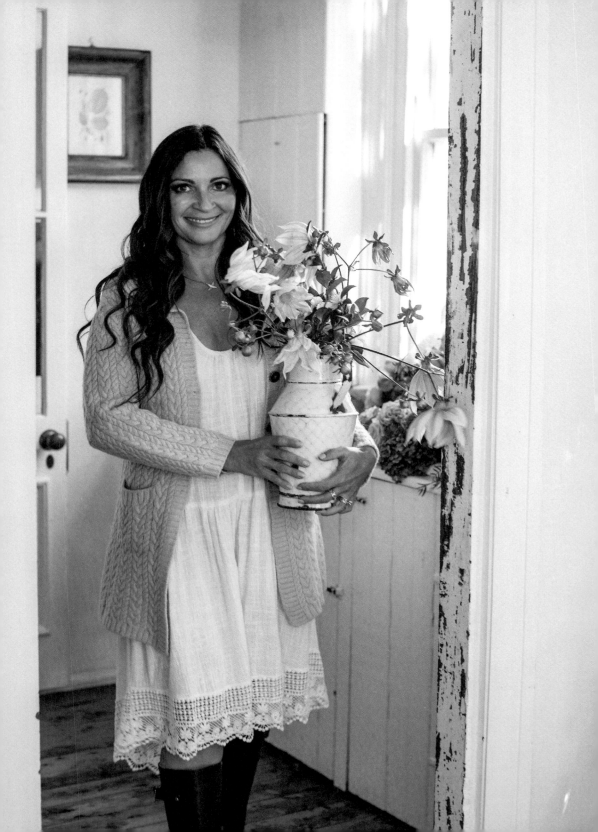

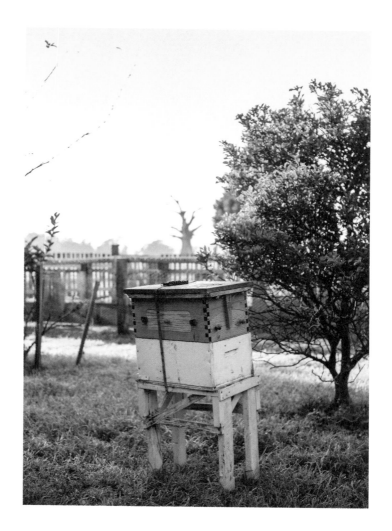

Now that you've rediscovered freedom and pleasure; created your personal food culture; cultivated your taste and flavour profiles; outfitted your kitchen pantry, fridge and freezer; chosen and consumed with purpose; shaped and personified a radio wave of supercharged embodiment; and connected the dots through commonsense eating and simple practices, it's time to invite an abundance of feel-good and nourishing recipes into your home and kitchen. Enjoy your supercharged life, and always be open and free to finding beauty and fulfilment in the everyday.

Notes

EAT

Nine winning flavour combos

p. 36

Increase your absorption of non-haem iron ...: Sean R. Lynch & James D. Cook, 'Interaction of vitamin C and iron', *Annals of the New York Academy of Sciences*, 1980, vol. 355, pp. 32–44, pdf.usaid.gov/pdf_docs/PNAAQ804.pdf.

This combination makes the perfect ....: Medijie Ang et al., 'Combining protein and carbohydrate increases postprandial insulin levels but does not improve glucose response in patients with type 2 diabetes', *Metabolism: Clinical and Experimental*, 2012, vol. 61, no. 12, pp. 1696–702.

Heart-healthy antioxidants found in foods ...: Brenda C. Davis & Penny M. Kris-Etherton, 'Achieving optimal essential fatty acid status in vegetarians: current knowledge and practical implications', *American Society for Clinical Nutrition*, 2003, vol. 78, no. 3, pp. 640S–66S, ajcn.nutrition.org/content/78/3/640S.full.

p. 37

Fat-soluble antioxidants like those found in tomatoes ...: Melody J. Brown et al., 'Carotenoid bioavailability is higher from salads ingested with full-fat than with fat-reduced salad dressings as measured with electrochemical detection', *American Journal of Clinical Nutrition*, 2004, vol. 80, no. 2, pp. 396–403, ajcn.nutrition.org/content/80/2/396.full.

The probiotics in fermented foods ...: Rosalind S. Gibson et al., 'Improving the bioavailability of nutrients in plant foods at the household level', *Proceedings of the Nutrition Society*, 2006, vol. 65, no. 2, pp. 160–68, www.cambridge.org/core/journals/proceedings-of-the-nutrition-society/article/div-classtitleimproving-the-bioavailability-of-nutrients-in-plant-foods-at-the-household-leveldiv/D1CC8CA0E2F3990871A5C7912619B8D7.

CONNECT Joining the dots

p. 269

As the Institute for the Psychology of Eating ...: Emily Rosen, 'Pleasure and metabolism', video, Institute for the Psychology of Eating, psychologyofeating.com/pleasure-and-metabolism-video-emily-rosen.

When people aiming to lower ...: 'A high-fat splurge', *Washington Post*, 24 November 1987, www.washingtonpost.com/archive/lifestyle/wellness/1987/11/24/a-high-fat-splurge/59daf5da-7357-4244-8993-178a721ef7ec/?utm_term=.5c2f2fe2fb5a.

Studies from Sweden and Thailand ...: L Hallberg et al., 'Iron absorption from Southeast Asian diets. II. Role of various factors that might explain low absorption', *American Journal of Clinical Nutrition*, 1977, vol. 30, no. 4, pp. 539–48, www.ncbi.nlm.nih.gov/pubmed/851082.

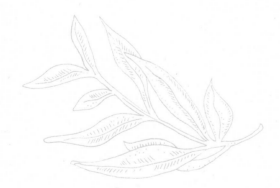

Index

These pictures are worth 61,000 words and my eternal gratitude.

Not forgetting my Murdoch Books team and Luisa, Sarah and Grace.

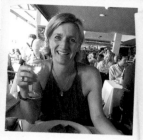
Cindy

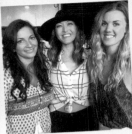
Candice and Emmily

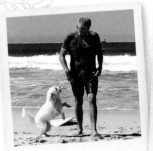
Justin

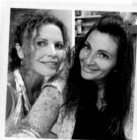
Lise

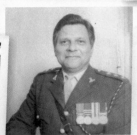
Dad

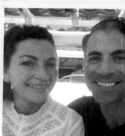
Dr Vincent Pedre

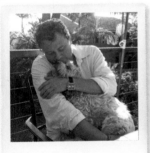
Simon

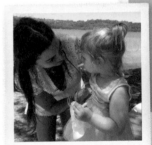
Brooklyn

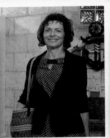
Lorraine

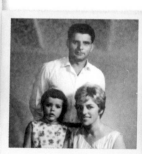
Mum

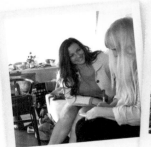
Diana

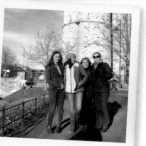
My UK family

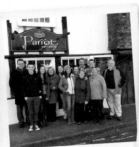
More UK family!

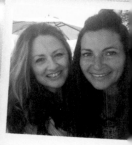
Lucy B

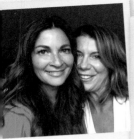

Michele

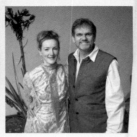

Georgie and Howard

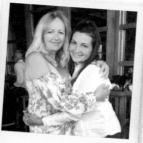

Jenny B

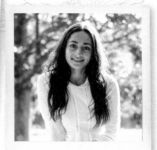

Tamsin

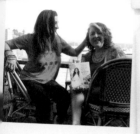

Aine the Irish Fairy

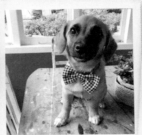

Oscar

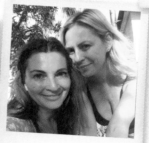

Juliet

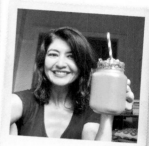

Brenda

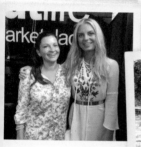

Vladia

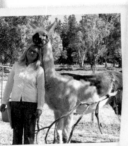

Margaret

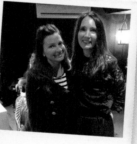

Pia

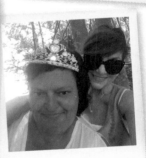

Roxy and Nicky

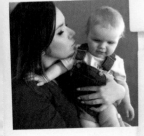

Arizona

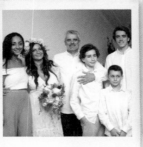

The Fam bam

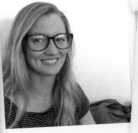

Jessica

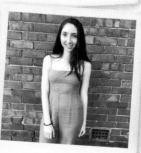

Toni

Published in 2019 by Murdoch Books,
an imprint of Allen & Unwin

Murdoch Books Australia
83 Alexander Street, Crows Nest NSW 2065
Phone: +61 (0) 2 8425 0100
Fax: +61 (0) 2 9906 2218
murdochbooks.com.au
info@murdochbooks.com.au

Murdoch Books UK
Ormond House, 26–27 Boswell Street
London WC1N 3JZ
Phone: +44 (0) 20 8785 5995
murdochbooks.co.uk
info@murdochbooks.co.uk

For Corporate Orders & Custom Publishing,
contact our Business Development Team
at salesenquiries@murdochbooks.com.au.

Publisher: Diana Hill
Editorial Manager: Katie Bosher
Design Manager: Madeleine Kane
Designer and Illustrator: Emily O'Neill
Additional typesetting: Transformer
Project Editor: Nicola Young
Photographer: Luisa Brimble
Stylist: Sarah O'Brien
Home Economists: Grace Campbell
and Dixie Elliott
Production Director: Lou Playfair

Text © Lee Holmes 2019
The moral rights of the author have been asserted.
Design © Murdoch Books 2019
Photography © Luisa Brimble 2019

Murdoch Books and the author wish to thank
Mark Whittaker and Amy Willesee of Willow Farm,
Berry, NSW for the use of their property.
willowfarmberry.com.au

A cataloguing-in-publication entry is available from
the catalogue of the National Library of Australia
at nla.gov.au.

ISBN 978 1 74336 637 0 Australia
ISBN 978 1 74336 639 4 UK

A catalogue record for this book is available
from the British Library.

Colour reproduction by Splitting Image
Colour Studio Pty Ltd, Clayton, Victoria
Printed by Leo Paper Group, China

IMPORTANT: Those who might be at risk from
the effects of salmonella poisoning (the elderly,
pregnant women, young children and those
suffering from immune deficiency diseases)
should consult their doctor with any concerns
about eating raw eggs.

The content presented in this book is meant
for inspiration and informational purposes only.
The purchaser of this book understands that
the author is not a medical professional, and
the information contained within this book is
not intended to replace medical advice or to
be relied upon to treat, cure, or prevent any
disease, illness, or medical condition. It is
understood that you will seek full medical
clearance by a licensed physician before making
any changes mentioned in this book. The author
and publisher claim no responsibility to any
person or entity for any liability, loss, or damage
caused or alleged to be caused directly or
indirectly as a result of the use, application,
or interpretation of the material in this book.

OVEN GUIDE: You may find cooking times
vary depending on the oven you are using.
For fan-forced ovens, as a general rule, set
the oven temperature to 20°C (70°F) lower
than indicated in the recipe.

MEASURES GUIDE: We have used
20 ml (4 teaspoon) tablespoon measures.
If you are using a 15 ml (3 teaspoon)
tablespoon add an extra teaspoon of the
ingredient for each tablespoon specified.

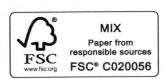